SEIZURE TRIGGERS

NEUROTOXINS AND EPILEPSY
IN ADULTS AND CHILDREN

*Learn to avoid possible seizures
as you read my personal story*

Second Edition

JUDI BRUNS

Published by:
What Elephant?

Second Edition 2023

Printed in the United States of America

Table of Contents

Table of Contents

I am grateful to:

All those that supported us through the Indiegogo campaign. This book would only be a continued thought if it were not for each and every one of them.

Every neurologist, physician, and medical worker who cares for their patients;

friends that helped through encouraging words and open ears;

my family, for their presence;

Mari-Carmen Gallego, for her support, guidance, ideas, and friendship throughout the years;

Ma, for her never-ending support in every adventure I started during my entire life and her loving encouragement to keep on writing;

and Dan, for everything, always.

Foreword

Epilepsy is a thief in the night. An epileptic seizure can suddenly happen to someone, steal peace, and then quite possibly instill fear and anguish into an otherwise happy life.

The theme of this book isn't so much about the lives of the people that wrote it. It is meant to bring to light triggers people may not be aware of as well as to convey knowledgeable ways to help deter a possible seizure. We share true life stories with correlative evidence in the hopes that those suffering from epilepsy, as well as those caring for them, can become more aware of neuro-toxic seizure triggers.

I am more in love with my wife than I knew could be possible after 30 years of marriage. She is an accomplished and organized magnetic resonance imaging (MRI) professional, a certified school teacher, an excellent snow skier, and an instructor, and her portfolio goes on academically. I feel it is fair to say that Judi has been sucker punched by challenging health conditions which started almost a year after we were married.

Judi is an over-achiever, fun-loving, thrill-seeking, quick-witted, and studious, as well as many other positive attributes one could add to her character or life resume. Over the years, through the hell and misery epilepsy can create, she has prevailed after each small or large setback to remain on a mission to continue forward toward her next goal. Not much of that goal-seeking made sense to me, as we were in the early years of our battle with epilepsy; and truthfully, not much of it makes much more sense to me now. But, I do believe that we must not stop believing in the future. This book is a mission and I feel honored to contribute a slice of content to it.

When Judi experienced her first grand-mal seizure, (this is the name I am used to calling it although it is now called a tonic-clonic seizure), I was there on an early Sunday morning in our bedroom in Hampton, Va. in the spring of 1992. I was in a state of shock, to say the least. I did not have any idea what had happened. So when it happened, I started a barbaric method of CPR, as I was dialing 911 on our landline. Shortly after this 60-90 second experience, which seemed much longer at the time, the paramedics showed up at our apartment on the 2nd floor. Based on her condition, they asked me if Judi had had a seizure. I responded, yes. She was then taken down on a gurney to the ER.

That seizure marked a new way of life for us. Each seizure created a new fork in the road or a drastic sudden change in our lifestyle. So after 30 years of choosing which direction to take with each seizure, I have reasoned to just take a straight line through the fork and strive to keep the focus on our only hope of power, love, and a sound mind. Christ Jesus was there every moment through it all, to guide us and offer us unending hope, love, and security.

Please realize that I do not always react to life's curve ball pitches the way I am spelling out here that we need to. Please forgive me for iterating the obvious to any of you as a reader or as a person dealing with these experiences, but I am reassuring and reminding myself as I write this how we need to live through and survive the challenges that epilepsy brings.

Epilepsy and all of its baggage carry a host of burdening emotions. This unpredictable illness can honestly drain everyone involved, whether it is you experiencing seizures or your loved one. If we, the caregiver, allow ourselves to become lackadaisical or beaten down emotionally, we are then of course less effective in helping the one we love. Epilepsy is scary for everyone involved, not just the person living with the condition. Patience as well as a persevering positive attitude is paramount and needs to be at the top of the prescription list, no matter the circumstance. I often fall short of this to be quite honest and open. I'm good at preaching the mantra, but I disappoint myself constantly. But again, fortunately, we all have a Savior that will never give up on any of us, ever. We just need to reset with every setback. Don't give up.

As the years went on, I found myself still freaking out during most of Judi's seizures that I was there to witness. I really did not need to call 911 again, but I still did during our second experience at the Omni Hotel in Gatlinburg on a spring morning in 1999. Again years later in the middle of another night after Judi had a major seizure, I went outside in the freezing cold of winter in my pajamas and just knelt down in the gravel driveway of one of our former homes in the beautiful mountains near Cherokee, N.C., and screamed to God. I do not remember what I was screaming, but I think I was screaming, "why?!"

How to Help

Care After a Seizure

I believe the most critical time that we as loving parents, spouses, family, and friends offer our assistance is after a seizure. Judi is very weak, groggy, unable to think straight, afraid, fragile, and vulnerable. In most of her awakenings after a seizure, she will get out of bed slowly, oftentimes needing my help. After a few minutes or maybe an hour or so, she will feel her tongue hurting, then ask me if she had a seizure. I try my best to nurture her in these delicate times of physical, mental, and emotional stress. Every tiny ounce of nourishment and dose of love that she can ingest and feel is so much needed to nourish and strengthen herself back emotionally.

I recommend keeping noisy electronics quiet during recovery. Try to take walks in nature and help the patient to take naps. Maybe also massage their neck, which has suffered an intense strain. Those journeys back to "normality" have seriously taken weeks! Although I really do not think Judi has ever regained all of what she lost with each seizure setback.

Take an Active Part

Taking an active part in the medical care of your loved one is pivotal. Judi has had a few great, caring, and patient neurologists over the 30 years of this battle and journey, and also unfortunately a neurologist that was lacking in patience. Judi is intelligent, she is inquisitive, she is concerned, caring, and kind in manner and emotion with people. She exhibits these traits during her check-ups with any neurologist or professional as well.

I accompanied Judi to 99% of her medical appointments in the early years. At one stretch of time, she had a neurologist that lacked the concern to listen and kindly answer a few simple questions Judi might have during visits. Judi's sister Jen, a Registered Nurse who was visiting us, accompanied Judi to a neurology check-up. After the appointment as they walked to the car, Jen mentioned, "You need a different neurologist." Physicians have it tough, but so do patients and loved ones that are legitimately concerned. The patient needs and deserves an advocate. One may just have to miss work to be able to stay with this person during doctor visits. Needless to say, we found another neurologist, even though we had to drive twice the distance.

We attended an epilepsy symposium in Nashville, Tennessee several years ago. There was one physician that spoke with a colleague for an hour regarding the fact that seizure medication can actually end up causing seizures due to toxic build-up in a patient's body.

I sometimes feel like I am my wife's doctor. I sincerely do not intend to seem arrogant with that statement or out of sorts in any way. It is just that there have been mistakes made over the years through the diagnosis, prognosis, and treatment process. Therefore, I try to use caution when I go into think-tank mode regarding my bride's health condition, but by the same token, I am not apprehensive or fearful to state my feelings based on my deductive reasoning and experiences with her.

In our early journey with epilepsy, I remember wondering about the chemicals Judi worked with in the X-ray department and my mother actually mentioned that concern to me as well. No physicians or neurologists mentioned neurotoxins to either of us throughout this epilepsy journey until Judi's brother Jim gave us a list of toxic products to steer clear of around the year 2002. Jim had acquired the list from a neurologist in Florida. This neurologist also mentioned to Jim, that if a neurologist did not mention these neuro-toxic products as a concern to a patient with epilepsy, then that patient probably needed to find a different neurologist.

Planning Ahead

As a spouse to a person with epilepsy, my coaching advice is to be proactive with a thought-through plan of where and how your loved one and yourself will spend your time together and apart throughout each day, week, and the rest of your life. I have met great people over the years that have shared pieces of their stories with me, regarding how they cared for their loved ones through illness and disease. A few of these stories were examples of how their bond of love grew stronger and some stories are tragic in how partners and even family members became embittered with negative emotions.

Every situation is different; every plan can change on a dime. It depends on lifestyle, in the home, out in nature, being adventurous, doing something new, or trying something different.

Judi still keeps Ativan with her no matter where she goes. Using it depends on the type and strength of the aura she has.

Think proactive for yourself. What will you be doing? What will you need? Whom will you be with? Will you be inside? Outside? Plan accordingly.

You cannot stop living your life.

Be Aware

There have been times when I have had to become an investigator. A couple of instances were when we had company stay with us for a few days. Our relatives and friends are aware of Judi's condition and the triggers outlined in this book. But just simply forget to think that the substances they have are not OK. Substances such as perfumes, colognes, haris sprays, and the like.

On another occasion, there was a smell that was driving Judi crazy in our home for weeks. She kept getting headaches and nausea from it. I was checking the bedroom that a relative had recently stayed in a few nights while visiting us. I was also checking underneath that bedroom in our basement for things that I could have brought in. I finally noticed a scented candle in the bedroom that the relative had been burning and then left after their stay. This candle even had a silicone-sealed lid, which I will intentionally add. I got rid of the candle, and things began to normalize.

Another occurrence was when we were storing some belongings for a relative under our pool table. Judi was experiencing aura after aura for weeks until I finally tore into the boxes of household belongings and found an opened can of Comet cleaner.

Please try to understand that I realize these case stories may seem redundant, but the subject point is really to try to convey a sense of how important and unconventional we need to think and be while assisting persons that are seizure prone; especially regarding public areas, new automobiles, new buildings, new clothing stores, etc. and consider any possible environments that may be releasing toxins.

We also know that PTSD can affect a person's mental and emotional health. Stress is also a well-known seizure trigger. Therefore, be aware of certain circumstances with friends, relatives, public places, noises, and any other situations that can trigger trauma, even while the person is sleeping.

Gardening

I am an avid gardener. I love it. The number one reason I grow a garden is to provide us with healthy, organic food. An example is leafy vegetables which can extract trace amounts of toxins from unhealthy soil. Synthetic fertilizers leave toxic residue in the soil. I try to grow potatoes, tomatoes, and other various veggies as much as possible for us. It is worth the extra cost and time invested. If you have the opportunity to garden, consider how much healthier it could be. Chapter 8 goes into more detail about diet.

Scuba Diving Story

Scuba Diving is a dangerous enough activity, without having epilepsy as an added concern. Here is just another crazy story of a few I might add, that Judi and I experienced in life.

We built and sold a few houses together before the financial plummet in 2009-10. So just before this housing crash, we sold our biggest prized home to a really great couple. Judi had always yearned to scuba dive and I was cool with doing it, except for the fact that it would cost money, and one other detail is the fact that Judi has epilepsy! We had sky miles to use and extra cash, so we flew to Florida to spend a few days in Pompano Beach.

Judi was so determined to scuba dive, and as we met and consulted with the diving crew and guides, the issue of epilepsy came up. Our guide explained quite patiently that it is really not a good idea for Judi to go scuba diving. Believe it or not, Judi is sort of starting to finally understand his point. So then my brain goes into this deductive reasoning mode or more appropriately stated, a deductive non-reasoning mode. I explain to her that she will still always want to go scuba diving and probably be somewhat down in the doldrums about it if she does not just go for it now. So we did. Not only that, but we ventured out into a lightning storm, the sky filled with black clouds. The guides were very professional, focused, and attentive. After our adventure, fun, and accomplishment, we decided together that we had accomplished that adventure goal, saw some sea life underwater, and that would wrap up our scuba diving escapades. I am not coaxing anyone with epilepsy to scuba dive. In retrospect, I am strongly advising against this practice. I am simply conveying one life story segment that was a goal for Judi. I really could have cared less at that point in my life if I went, but I knew what it meant to her, even with the risk.

The point here is that sometimes we take chances in life. Having epilepsy can be extremely limiting, especially for someone that does things...adventurous things whenever possible. Life is what we make it. Some things may be worth taking a risk on, and some things are just not. This is a decision that you and your loved one make together. Also, go ahead and add the doctor to that decision process.

The Good

What can we glean from our trials? Here is a story that helped me see beyond our own personal difficulties.

Judi and I were visiting her mom at an assisted living apartment complex. We were outside talking and we watched a woman walking to her apartment. We knew this woman also had epilepsy and she lived alone. There was no one else around, and I observed this lady start to have a seizure. I quickly stepped up my pace towards her and caught her in my arms and gently brought her as softly as I could to the ground. Judi and her mom mentioned that they had no idea what she was doing. It wasn't a tonic-clonic seizure, but I could just tell that it was a type of seizure. I guess I was extra sensitive and aware of her condition due to the many episodes I had dealt with over the years with Judi. In cases like this, I can say that I feel sort of blessed that I was able to assist that woman.

We can't always understand why we go through the trials we go through. But they can make us stronger. I am married to a woman with epilepsy and it changed the course of our life. I'd like to think I have grown through this. Judi and I have also grown closer together through this. We can of course become stronger from trials, and I pray that I may continue to be strong for my beautiful wife.

Final Words

Judi actually battled about whether or not to write this book. She and I decided together that this book may seem on the surface that it is about us and our story, but we both just want the book to have a purpose to help others. We have our family, our Foster Church family in Asheville, NC, as well as our skiing colleagues who have all supported us so much with prayers, love, gifts, and emotional support. Without this support that actually came from God through all of these caring people, we wouldn't have the zeal and resilience to strive forward and bring all of this together. God will continue with us, as this journey and battle go on. God has been with us all along. He is there for you as well. To have the sustaining power to keep on keepin' on, we just try to keep our eyes on Jesus.

My small story account is sincerely meant so that hopefully some readers will glean some value and plan routes for their journey toward a more fulfilling and safer lifestyle. To improve the lives of the individuals suffering from seizures as well as the lives of individuals caring for them.

Dan Bruns, Judi's husband

Introduction

The Bomb

My life as a young adult before epilepsy was the bomb. Really... I was athletic and active. I could eat anything I wanted, and usually did. I drank Pepsi, coffee, and Gatorade. I ate M&M's, Twix bars, and Doritos; all in moderation of course. I washed my hair with any shampoo I thought smelled good and used lotions and creams that seemed to fill the room. I loved using sweet-smelling perfumes that made me feel beautiful. I loved painting my nails and toenails in the summer and wearing cute sandals that showed off my handwork of little flowers and hearts. I was able to drive anywhere I wanted and fill up the car with gas without a second thought.

Walking into stores was a norm for me. I didn't much care for shopping, but it was something that I needed to do. Walking down aisles and admiring clothes, shoes, and perfumes was something I did whenever I wanted. Going shopping with my mom and sister made it more fun than going by myself. Then we would head to a restaurant and enjoy some freshly cooked food and enjoy talking about our day.

Special times I may have taken for granted.

But then, when I turned twenty-four and shortly after I got married, a bomb of a different kind showed up in my life.

My first seizure.

I share my story in Chapter 2, but for now, I'll say it came as a surprise, to say the least.

What did I know about seizures? Where did my history begin? I remember when I was about five years old in the middle of the night, I was awakened by a weird noise coming from the living room. I peeked around the corner to see my mom "wrestling" with my brother on the couch. He was kicking around. She had a wooden spoon in her hand and was trying to get it in his mouth. What in the world was this all about?!

My mom noticed me out of the corner of her eye and yelled at me to get back to my room and in bed. Like I was going to just go back to sleep after witnessing that! Yes, it bothered me, and no, I will never forget it. It was like a tattoo that never seemed to go away, no matter how many times I feverishly tried to scrub it out of my mind.

I later learned that this was the protocol for someone having a seizure during these earlier years. To hold the tongue down so they wouldn't swallow it or choke to death. This, by the way, is archaic and advised against. There is absolutely no way that someone can swallow their tongue. Thank God for progressing forward, for knowledge, research, and epilepsy awareness in the medical field.

Epilepsy is said to be both inherited and acquired. Meaning, it can be passed down through the genes of the parents, but it can also occur as a "new" condition when cells are dividing. I guess it just decided to hit me at a later age for no known or apparent reason. There is some heredity of seizures in my family. My brother has had epilepsy ever since he was about eleven years old. He was immediately put on Dilantin. This was about fifty years ago, when there were not many drugs to choose from, and he is still taking them. For the most part, it has controlled his seizures. But being on medication like that for that many years has got to take its toll on his body. Since I mentioned my brother, I would like to share something that my brother does. He controls his seizures. I mean he can stop one from coming on. He tried to explain to me, how he focuses on an object and forces his mind to think in a new way, contrary to what he is seeing. It was hard for me to totally understand what he was saying, but the point was, that it works for him. He can literally stop a seizure with his vision and thought process. It may sound odd, but I can relate in a small way. When I do get an aura, I try to engage my mind. I may try to have a conversation with Dan, or talk to someone on the phone, or I may even talk aloud about something detailed. I get my mind off of the aura and engage it elsewhere. Honestly, I don't know if this actually stops my seizures, but I will say that often, the aura does not progress into a full-blown grand-mal (tonic-clonic) seizure. I will continue throughout this book to call a grand mal seizure a tonic-clonic seizure as that is what it is now called (even though the name grand mal is still continually used).

Now, I am not a general practitioner, a neurologist, or a physiologist. I am a ski instructor, an inventor, an entrepreneur, a wife to my nurturing husband (a work in progress), a step-mom to two wonderful young adults, a Tia (auntie in Spanish) to some pretty awesome nieces and nephews, a grandma to an amazing granddaughter, a daughter to a supportive mom, a sister to some loving sisters and brothers, and a mom to my service dog Violet (more about her later in the book). But just like my brother, I also have epilepsy. An illness you cannot see, as all disabilities are not visible. Notice I said I have epilepsy last of all. I refuse to let it define me because it is only a part of me, and not who I am.

Epilepsy is defined as a neurological disorder characterized by recurrent seizures, which cause blackouts accompanied by full-blown tonic-clonic (aka grand mal) seizures with convulsions or absence (petit mal) seizures that are barely noticeable at all.

There is no known common cause, and there is no known cure.

Epilepsy has been around for thousands of years, but all we can do is treat it; hopefully, stop a seizure with medications and try to minimize our side effects. While medical research hasn't yet uncovered *why* epilepsy exists, we understand that what can trigger a seizure in one person may not affect another. For instance, many smells trigger my seizures, but they may not affect others at all.

So, why is epilepsy so hard to control? Why hasn't the medical field found a cure? Why is epilepsy such an enigma?

I cannot answer those questions. I can only share what I went through, what I have learned, the things that triggered my seizures, and what I did and still do to avoid a seizure, and hope and pray that it helps you or someone you love.

Who Has Epilepsy?

It is estimated that over sixty-five million people worldwide suffer from epilepsy (it was fifty million when I started this book!). Epilepsy is the fourth most common neurological problem, with only migraine, stroke, and Alzheimer's disease occurring more frequently. According to the Epilepsy Foundation, epilepsy isn't rare; it's more than twice as common in the US as cerebral palsy, muscular dystrophy, multiple sclerosis, and cystic fibrosis *combined*.[1] Yes, combined!

Some quick statistics about epilepsy (currently):

- Sixty-five million people worldwide suffer from epilepsy.
- Roughly 1:10 will have a seizure sometime in their lifetime.
- Over a lifetime, 1:26 individuals in the U.S. will be diagnosed with epilepsy.
- Each year, 150,000 Americans are diagnosed with epilepsy.
- It is estimated that 5 million people worldwide are diagnosed with epilepsy each year.
- At least 1 million people in the United States have uncontrolled (drug-resistant) epilepsy.

---

[1] "Facts about Seizures and Epilepsy," Epilepsy Foundation, https://www.epilepsy.com/learn/about-epilepsy-basics/facts-about-seizures-and-epilepsy.

- 1 out of every 1000 people with epilepsy dies from SUDEP each year.

These stats are changing so fast, I cannot keep up. As edits were made to my first edition bringing about this second edition, the numbers increased dramatically. These numbers are shocking and heartbreaking. Seizures in children, young adults, middle aged adults, and seniors. Epilepsy shows no prejudice. No bias. No favoritism.

Historical People who Had Epilepsy

Records show that epilepsy has been affecting people at least since the beginning of recorded history. Throughout ancient history, this disease was thought to be a spiritual condition. In Babylonian times, they attributed seizures to being possessed by evil spirits. The ancient Greeks, however, thought of epilepsy as a form of spiritual possession and associated the condition with genius and the divine. It was referred to as a falling sickness and thought of as a Sacred Disease. Due to his fame as a conqueror in battle, Alexander the Great was thought to have a sense of divinity with his seizures. Other great men in history such as Julius Caesar, Hercules, Socrates, and Napoleon Bonaparte had epilepsy as well. Defining epilepsy, its causes, its meaning, and its effects, was elusive, to say the least.

When did the ideas of epilepsy and its meaning start to evolve? Roughly around the fourth century BC. Hippocrates was born around 460 BC on the island of Kos, Greece. He became known as the founder of medicine and was regarded as the greatest physician of his time. The whole idea of spirits, whether evil or good, was not favored by Hippocrates. He soon rejected the idea that epilepsy was caused by spirits, but rather a treatable medical problem originating in the brain. His view, however, was not accepted at the time. Not until at least the seventeenth century, evil spirits continued to be blamed. In ancient Rome, people did not drink or eat with the same pottery used by someone who had seizures.

Here is a cool historic fact. To detect epilepsy, ancient physicians would light a piece of gagate (jet, a precursor to coal) and its smoke would trigger a seizure. I found this amazing! This sounds like a seizure triggered by a smell as I have! What I also find interesting, but less endearing, is that although medicine has brought us incredible knowledge about epilepsy, a thread of stigma has been maintained throughout history. Good spirits, bad spirits, brain conditions. This stigma can and has affected people economically, socially, mentally, physically, and culturally. Even now, in some countries, people in some areas believe that those with epilepsy are cursed. Marriages could even be annulled due to seizures not just long ago! This stigma still exists today. Maybe not to the same degree as in our history, but it is still there.

Let's consider other well-known individuals—writers, athletes, entertainers, etc.—who have lived with a seizure disorder (or so it is thought) at least at one point of time in their lives. Individuals such as Vincent van Gogh, Michelangelo, Edgar Allen Poe, Albert Einstein, and Thomas Edison. There is some debate as to whether they had epilepsy, but based on what we know, we can assume they had some type of neurological challenge.

Florence Griffith Joyner, nicknamed Flo-Jo, was an American Olympian. She died in 1998 from an epileptic seizure (now known as SUDEP, or Sudden Unexpected Death in Epilepsy). What's awesome is her quote: "When someone tells me I can't do anything, I'm just not listening anymore."

Susan Boyle, known for her remarkable rendition of "I Dreamed a Dream" on *Britain's Got Talent*, struggled with epilepsy and is quoted as saying: "To anyone who has a dream, I say follow that dream. You are never too old. It is never too late."

Theodore Roosevelt, the twenty-sixth president of the United States, had epilepsy. He is quoted as saying: "Courage is not having the strength to go on; it is going on when you don't have the strength." Wow, just wow!

I need to mention Danny Glover, the actor well-known for his performance as a Los Angeles Police Sergeant in the "Lethal Weapon" movies. He has epilepsy and suffered from seizures during a twenty-year period of his life. He is an advocate for epilepsy and supports the Epilepsy Foundation working to bring awareness of epilepsy and its many issues. I read that he has outgrown his seizures. I realize this is possible for some people. I can't say too much about how we can outgrow a seizure. I guess our bodies just stop causing havoc due to possible underlying issues...or maybe it just gets tired. It is definitely more common for kids to outgrow a seizure than it is for adults, but hey, we can always hope it can happen to us as well. What a blessing for him.

I recently read that Harriet Tubman had epilepsy. Her epilepsy was due to a traumatic brain injury when a slave owner struck her in the head. Have you watched the movie "Harriet"? If not, consider taking the time to watch this truly inspiring movie. What respect and awe I have for her. Talk about a woman that made change happen. What stamina, guts, and perseverance! All that she did, even while dealing with epilepsy.

Although seizures can be disruptive, they do not have to stop us from living and enjoying our lives in some way. We can live well and find success in combination with the many challenges of this disease. I realize one's definition of success may differ from someone else's. How you define success is where the mark is. Let each of us hit the mark that we have for ourselves, not someone else's.

Neurotoxins May Cause Epilepsy

Could neurotoxins actually trigger a seizure? The quick answer? Yes! Dan and I can attest to this. We had the opportunity to speak at length with a medical doctor several years ago while I was performing volunteer medical interpreting services at a clinic. We also believe that neurotoxins play a much larger role in seizure activity than many realize. We are obviously surrounded by toxins! Toxins are found in our bodies, on our bodies, in what we eat, in the air we breathe, what we put on our hair, and in what we smell. I will provide a list of toxins that directly triggered a seizure for me in Chapter 3.

Most of the toxins I talk about caused a direct, 100% correlative proof, five-second-later tonic-clonic seizure. Some were auras resulting in other types of seizures, migraines, and other varying neurological responses. Depending on the actual trigger, my response would be different. Sometimes the resulting seizure had a quick onset, other times, it took hours, and still other times not until the next day.

Of course, **we are all so different**. My triggers may not be your triggers, but if avoiding or striving to avoid toxins could help you avoid having a seizure, wouldn't you like to know more about them? Whether you are reading this book for yourself, a spouse, a family member, or a friend, the information you find here could be very helpful. If you discover that these triggers do not induce a seizure in you, thank God! Yet, just because you may not react right away to toxins, don't be fooled as to the harm they can have on us as humans and on our environment. There are many things that we can do to help avoid having a seizure and hopefully at the same time avoid becoming another statistic.

The Frustrating Aspects of Epilepsy

I suppose the hard part is that epilepsy is like an untold story. The whole "secrecy" of it all. You can't see it from the outside. Unless someone has a seizure right in front of you, you may never know they suffer silently. In my opinion, it's an overlooked, serious illness. There is research being done on it, but it remains an enigma. Its causes vary immensely, and how it is demonstrated through people varies even more. The thing that triggers a seizure in one person may not trigger a seizure in someone else. Maybe that's why I feel epilepsy just hangs out there on the sidelines of a true medical condition, and its awareness is even more so. How can scientists anchor a ship that is guided by ebb and flow?

I feel kind of left out and I feel others may as well. Only within the past few years have I regularly seen epilepsy as a condition you hear about or read about. Thirty years ago, epilepsy was not even an illness to mark on medical forms at the doctor's office. It just wasn't there. I had to write it in, and sometimes, I just didn't. I was too embarrassed. Where was the concern that epilepsy is a real condition, a real disease to be aware of? I am thankful that it is finally getting the attention it deserves. Doctors need to know that we have epilepsy, and we need to tell them.

One of the most frustrating aspects of having seizures is their unpredictability. They can occur due to so many different factors, with some having absolutely no correlation. Triggers are so erratic and difficult to pinpoint. They have no standardized means of telling if a seizure will result from a certain trigger or not. Take a tack for instance; if you stick yourself with a tack, you will bleed. This is a fact. One action caused a reaction. Problem solved: don't stick yourself with a tack and you won't bleed. Triggers for seizures are not black and white. They're not even grey. If one person has a seizure due to flickering lights, the next person may not be affected at all. This of course makes it a huge challenge to pinpoint triggers and offer sound medical advice. The most important thing I can say is that every person is different. Every response to a possible trigger varies as greatly as each person varies. This of course applies to the treatment as well. What works for one patient, can send another to the hospital, as one medication did to me; that story is a little later. Knowledge is potential power. Let's share our knowledge with each other and be empowered with greater resistance against epilepsy.

What I find invigorating is the fact that epilepsy is becoming known. I mean, I'm glad people are seeing it as a real disease and not an illness that has to be hidden. I also love the fact that our world is becoming more and more aware of the toxins that exist in so many man-made substances. I love that alternative healthier products are more readily available to us than they were twenty years ago. Just knowing you can easily purchase natural organic cleaners versus toxic cleaners is inspiring. Manufacturers are making changes to their products, praise God! Isn't it time for more of us to make changes in the products that we use?

Effects

I mentioned this varying thread of stigma that has remained throughout time. Let's face it, it is still there. I believe it exists with seizures, epilepsy, and other neurological disorders as well. What about the word *epileptic*? I think that word carries even more stigma. We can't deny its existence, but there are things we can do to help us overcome it.

I personally think it is an embarrassing illness. I do. I won't lie. I am embarrassed I have epilepsy. There I said it. You see, it's not just about seizures. Yeah, they are bad enough. But it's so much more. Maybe you get it. Maybe you are dealing with what some of us deal with every day. Seizures. Now add dizziness, fatigue, memory loss; loss of independence and the ability to drive; having to rely on others to go anywhere, questioning your abilities, being self-conscious; and of course living with the fear of having a seizure in public. It's easier to tell someone you have diabetes or arthritis. But telling someone you have seizures? I don't think so. We hide it. We prefer to live behind our self-created walls, which we may not even know we're creating.

Many people who suffer from epilepsy, I've found, have similar emotions. Scared to have a seizure in public, afraid to have a seizure at home. Wondering if you took your meds because you cannot remember. Apprehensive to start a new job, continually forgetting things, wondering what will trigger your next seizure, afraid of possible side effects from the medications, wondering if your symptoms are rare or if others have them too. Does anyone else suffer from neuropathy? Headaches? Nausea? Bad mood swings? Thyroid changes? Worried about pregnancy? When can I drive again? Am I eating enough? Am I eating too much? Am I sleeping too much? Am I sleeping enough? Are visual changes normal? Is brain fog normal? Does a sore tongue mean I had a seizure? Is speech delay normal? Am I the only one that feels this depressed? Anxious? Scared? Why hasn't the medical field pinpointed my seizure triggers? I mean, we can send a man to the moon, can't we? What can help me avoid triggers that could possibly lessen the probability of having a seizure? What are my triggers? Why doesn't my doctor know? What don't I know? What am I going to do about my epilepsy?

Although I do not answer all of the above questions, I pray you can find some answers to many of them in this book. I have been dealing with seizures for thirty years and have been able to make direct links between my seizures to certain triggers. Triggers that are often not talked about or known. For me at least, I have made many changes in my life to hopefully avoid my discovered triggers. Maybe you can too.

Should epilepsy define us? No matter how hard it gets, no matter the trials it brings, no matter the stigma we face, and no matter the debilitating emotions that flood us daily, it still does not have the power to control us. It does not have the power to dictate how our lives are to be lived. It cannot dictate who we are. Don't give epilepsy that much power!

We decide that. *God, help us as we take control of our lives: Give us fortitude and determination to hold our heads up high and fight. Better yet, fight for us, Lord, as at times our strength can be almost nonexistent. We struggle. We give up. We fall short. Pick us up, Lord, as you have done for those before us. We are purple warriors!*

Understanding Triggers

What exactly is a trigger? A trigger is a factor or a situation that can bring on a seizure in someone that does or does not have epilepsy. As I mentioned earlier, 1 in 100 people will have a seizure at some point in their lives, but this does not mean that they will develop epilepsy. It may be that one and only time. The cause of a seizure is not the same thing. A cause may be an accident, a brain tumor, or a genetic tendency for example. Triggers themselves are the actual factors such as flashing lights or burning Teflon, as examples. I believe that the line between a cause and a trigger can

11

sometimes be hard to differentiate, especially when it comes to alcohol for example. Alcohol can be the cause of someone having seizures, but can also be a trigger for someone. However, I'm sure you get the point. The "trigger" is what triggers/sets off the brain to react to a particular stimulus resulting in a seizure.

With the help of my husband, Dan, we have spent the last thirty years learning about my triggers. Unfortunately, by trial and error. Dan can remember details like the color of the scrubs the nurse was wearing when I had my first seizure! He's pretty handy to have around; he's my rock.

We have learned that my seizures are primarily triggered by smells. One of the cranial nerves, the olfactory nerve, has the dutiful job of transmitting information relating to smell to the brain for processing. These smells can be beautiful aromas from roses and lavender fields as well as dangerous poignant environmental toxins that exist in our world today. Toxins may not have been as prevalent in the past as they are now. No wonder one in twenty-six people in the US will develop epilepsy at some point in their lifetime.

My smell-induced triggers fall under a type of epilepsy called reflex epilepsy. I go over this in a little more detail in Chapter 3. I learned this through my research. My family physician didn't tell me this and neither did my neurologist. It's just that reflex epilepsy and smell-induced seizures are not commonly known or recognized.

Through it all, I have kept notes and would like to share them. Maybe you or someone you know could benefit from knowing these possible triggers.

There must be more knowledge about triggers. For this reason, I am sharing my journey—to advocate for epilepsy awareness, to possibly help the 3.4 million people nationwide and the more than 65 million globally who struggle with epilepsy and its effects both physical and mental.

Be Your Own Investigator

Because epilepsy is so difficult to treat, we need to be our own best investigators.

Not our own doctors, our own investigators. There are many loving, caring neurologists, epileptologists, and other physicians out there. I love them and thank God for their care, knowledge, and expertise. They are our heroes. They keep us going and do the best they can. But, often, they miss possible triggers. They know how to regulate our medication, but they cannot regulate how we live our lives. We need to step in and take a proactive step toward our care.

To be our own best investigator, we need to know what is going on with our bodies. It's too easy to just take a pill. We need to do more.

When you do have a seizure, think about everything, and I do mean everything. Think about things just before the seizure, days before even, and document it. Write it down because you will forget (just like me):

- What was I doing when the aura hit me?
- What was happening just prior to my seizure?
- What were people doing around me?
- Where was I?
- Were there toxic fumes in the area?
- Had I smelled anything odd?
- How was my health that day?
- Had I eaten right?
- Did I eat right yesterday?
- What did I drink?
- Did I drink enough water today?
- Did I drink enough water yesterday?

- What happened yesterday?
- How is my mental health?
- Am I over-tired?
- Am I sick?
- Was I angry?
- Was I hungry?

You get the idea. We need to investigate what could have possibly been a trigger. Seek to identify it. And seek to avoid it in the future.

We are entering a new phase in epilepsy treatment. Self-care. Self-awareness. Not self-treatment, but self-knowledge to aid our neurologists and epileptologists with the care that we receive. It's not just them writing a script to hopefully control our seizures. It's us taking an active role in the management of our seizures.

What This Book Aims to Do

I am a very "get to the point" kind of person. I grew up in New England and never quite understood the Southern way of "sugarcoating" things. As you read this book, I might come across as harsh, demanding, and strict. I do say things like, don't do this, don't do that, and suck it up. In my humble opinion, life is too short to beat around the bush, and our illness can be too debilitating to sugarcoat things. Just remember, I love all my purple warrior family. Be strong and read on.

This book does not aim to answer all the questions I've already brought up above, but it does aim to tell you that you are not alone. You have a family of fighters that have gone through or are going through, the very things you are fighting. All the thoughts, emotions, and questions that you are entangled with, someone else is entangled in them as well.

This book aims to inform you of seizure triggers out there in the world that may have never crossed your mind as being a possible trigger. Also, this book aims to encourage you to make lifestyle changes that may lessen the possibility of having seizures.

We are purple warriors, and we just don't give up. We keep on fighting.

I know it's not easy. Having seizures and the fear of having a seizure at any point and time in my life can be debilitating. But I believe that many of you reading this book can learn to overcome these debilitating, controlling feelings. I believe that we have within our ability the means of learning certain triggers and avoiding those triggers to live a more normal life each day. Yes, normal is a relative word.

I pray that this book helps you to learn a way in which others can get to know you. I believe you are a wonderful person and when others truly get to know you, then both you and I will be blessed. One of the most important means of a joyful life is the relationships that we form—relationships with our family, our spouse, our friends, our church family, our business acquaintances,

15

and even strangers. One word can change one's life so dramatically. Live life to the fullest; that is what God created you to do.

Who You Are

Here's an exercise. Write down the type of person you are. Write down who you are, deep down inside, and what you are like. Do not write all the bad stuff. We all have bad stuff in our lives. Write down the attributes that people can look at and admire. Take the time and search deep. You may even need to get help from a close family member or a good friend that can help you look past the negative that we all have. It's sad that we can quickly rattle off tons of our bad qualities, and struggle with naming one or two good things about ourselves. Either way, write them down and add more to the list whenever you can.

Once you have done this, read it every single day. Read it until you convince yourself that you are a good person, full of promise, full of something that you can bless others with. No, this is not easy for some of us.

Don't let seizures and epilepsy define you! You are God's child, a prince, a princess! You are fearfully and wonderfully made (Psalms 139:14). The Hebrew translation of fearfully is *heart-felt interest, respect,* and *great reverence.* Wonderfully can be translated as *unique* and *set apart.* We are individually set apart for a special purpose, regardless of what this world throws at us. God has a heartfelt interest in each one of us. Wow, that really personalizes it for me!

Chapter 1
My Life Before Epilepsy

A Smart and Determined Girl

Do you know that sweet little girl sitting on the side of the classroom with messy hair and dirty jeans? That was me. The quiet one. The insecure one. The mischievous little smarty pants one. I was a smart kid doing quite well in the first grade, better than the average student at that level. I'm not tooting my own horn, just mentioning this to say that people with epilepsy can be and are smart! One day, one of the teachers pulled me aside. "Judi, we would like to move you up to a higher-level class. We just need you to take this test."

They handed me a piece of paper with some pictures and a few questions on it. Glancing over the questions, I smirked and said to myself, "This is easy." I knew every single answer in less than five seconds. For some odd reason, I sat there acting like I didn't know the answers and fiddling around with my pencil. The teacher came over and asked me what was wrong and why I wasn't answering the questions. I looked up undoubtedly with a pitiful look on my face and said, "Because I don't know the answers."

What? Why on earth did I say that? As an adult, I can look back and sum up my entire childhood. I was purely seeking attention. Growing up in a family of five, I was number four. Two older brothers, an older sister, and a younger sister. Of the three youngest kids, us girls, I was the middle child. Was there a "middle-child syndrome" that affected me? Maybe. My life growing up was difficult. We lived in Fairhaven, Massachusetts. My mom was a single mom doing the best she could trying to raise us kids.

So, that first-grade test was to determine my entire life's future or at least affect it in some way. I was left in the "slow" class.

That's what it was called back in the day. The gifted classes, and the slower learning classes. We kids knew the difference. I am sure it affected us in so many ways.

But once I hit the fifth grade, they moved me to the gifted class every day for math. Several of the kids in the gifted class would come over to the slower class, and I was the only one to go to the gifted class. Did I excel? Yes, and had the highest grade in that math class to boot! I am thankful that our education system has at least improved in many ways since then. No doubt, we still have a long way to go.

Go-getter Spirit

I really had a go-getter attitude from a young age. I had my first paying job when I was about seven years old. I made fifty cents a day emptying trash cans after school. There were two long (nearly never-ending) wings in my elementary school. The janitor paid me twenty-five cents a wing to empty each of the trash cans from each room into a big rolling trash cart I pushed down the empty hall. I don't specifically remember asking the janitor if he needed help, but I was not one to turn down any amount of money. I do know that he offered me the job when he saw me hanging around the halls after all the kids had already left.

I stuck around there because I was bullied. Guess I just didn't quite fit in. I was afraid to walk home as I knew I would get beat up. Working for the janitor gave all the kids time to go home and at the same time gave me a peaceful walk home. Sad, but true. This unfortunate time in my life had a good point. I made money. I liked the fact that I could stop at the small corner convenience store and buy five little red candied fish (don't buy these now, by the way; they have red dye, which can be a seizure trigger) for five cents and save the leftover forty-five cents toward a bike.

Things pretty much stayed this way for several years. When my stepdad came onto the scene, I was in the third or fourth grade. At around ten years old, I secured my own paper route and started passing out about fifty daily papers in the neighborhood. Each day after school, I would throw that pack of papers on my skinny little shoulders and start my delivery on my walk toward home. Rain, sunshine, snow, ice, it didn't seem to stop the paper company from making papers and it didn't seem to stop me. Now, this was good money. I want to say I made about $10 a week. My parents had this very cool deal where they would pay for half of the things that I wanted. Not necessities like clothes and food, but fun things like games, a baseball glove, a bat, a basketball, etc. My mind was set on a bike: Man, would this help as far as carrying that pack of newspapers! And I only had to pay half for it! My money jar was slowly filling up. The best days on the paper route job were when my stepdad was home from fishing trips because he would let me sit on the back of his station wagon and tailgate my entire route. I would jump off and run from house to house with a rolled-up newspaper in my hand. I loved it when he was home.

An Active, Athletic Lifestyle

I enjoyed every sport imaginable. I joined the boys' baseball team simply because there wasn't a girls' team at that time. I was the only girl on my team, and I didn't care. I do think there was only one other girl in the entire league. I played baseball for a couple of years and loved it! Basketball was the next sport I jumped right into. I joined a girls' basketball camp that my Uncle John helped me get into and I loved it. I found myself learning with the best of the best. I worked hard and excelled even though I was one of the shortest girls playing. I kept playing basketball, and in high school, I became a point guard and MVP (most valuable player) for several years.

I continued staying very active. I ran, biked, and played any kind of sport that was available to me. In college, I continued my active lifestyle. I went snow skiing once and water skiing a few times. I got good at racquetball and loved learning new sports. I took college seriously. I was never into the whole party scene and never went out drinking. Well, before a friend reading this throws me under the bus, I did go out one time. I had one drink, got sick, and never drank again. I thought it was the stupidest thing anyone could do. I would rather focus on my classes. I was paying for my schooling. I felt no desire to waste money. I was working so hard to do what I was set out to do. I loved to get the highest grade in every single one of my classes. Not to say this happened, but I tried.

Even though I knew I wanted to be in college, I was still unsure what exactly I wanted to do with my life. Only because a friend was taking radiology classes at a two-year college in Kettering, Ohio, I thought I would, too. (I really show my insecurities again here.)

This friend, by the way, ended up being my sister-in-law. I met my husband at her wedding. I had to march with one of the groom's brothers. More of that story later.

A Death in the Family

During my last year of the radiology program, my stepdad had a sudden, unexpected heart attack and passed away. This happened during Christmas break, just a few months prior to my graduation with an A.S. degree in radiology. He was living in Florida, and I flew down there to join the family for Christmas. I arrived on December 19. My mom and little sister had all they owned in a car moving from Massachusetts to Florida to join him. They arrived on December 20. He died the next morning.

I had a hard time getting things back together after that. Oh, the curve balls life throws at you. I really didn't know how to deal with things. My mom, now alone with my sister, did the best she could. I felt like I needed to help, but how? I failed the radiology program. What? Me? I do not accept failure. How in the world could this have happened? I guess I had a really hard time getting my head back into the game after that Christmas break. What do I do now? Where do I go? I usually ran from my failures, so I did. I applied to a four-year college in Michigan. I settled on architecture and loved it. Unfortunately, I couldn't afford a four-year college. So, I went back to finish my radiology degree. I went back only because a friend did. He had failed out, too, but decided to finish and I just went with him. Once again, my insecurities blocked my own decision-making process. I only had to repeat the last semester and fulfill my obligation with a clinical rotation in the hospital. I might add here that all through college, I worked three jobs. I worked in the kitchen at the hospital, Pizza Hut, and Skyline Chili. I was working and studying all the time.

Meeting Dan

Immediately after graduation, I enrolled in the Magnetic Resonance Imaging (MRI) program and became a certified MRI technologist half a year later. As a technologist, I would operate a machine that uses magnetic resonance to scan and create detailed images of internal organs. Not like you all don't know about MRI as I am sure each of you has had your fair share and then some. I feel fortunate that I had the opportunity to study MRI. It has been a huge blessing to me as I was able to read the studies quite well and ask my neurologist the needed questions.

This was about the time that I got married to my friend's brother-in-law. Here is the quick story on that.

When I was attending college in Michigan, my friend asked me to be one of her bridesmaids. When the time came, I drove back to Kettering, Ohio, for the wedding. She matched me with the groom's shortest brother, Dan.

We were all gathered around for the rehearsal, but no Dan was in sight. I was told he was working but should be here soon. The entire night, no Dan to be seen. I faked motions of taking his arm as he would soon lead me up the steps to stand with the other bridesmaids. Still no Dan. The next morning, I was wondering where this Dan guy was so I could at least introduce myself. The wedding party has another quick get-together in the church before the ceremony begins. Once again, no Dan is to be found. I resigned myself to seeing the guy after I walked down the aisle.

Finally, as the ceremony commenced, I held my flowers and started down the church aisle. Good, I could see him down there now, I thought, at least I won't be alone. When I was close enough

21

to see his eyes, my entire stomach flipped upside down. Oh, my goodness, I was smitten. He was handsome, dark-complexioned from working out in the sun all day, and he had these killer blue eyes. Tall, dark, and handsome? I'll settle for short, dark, and handsome. I tried to shrug off my excitement and hope he didn't notice. The rest of the evening was like a fairy tale. He was polite, caring, and attentive, and danced with me more than once.

At the end of the reception, I had to head back to Michigan. I jumped in the car with some friends ready to go, but I wanted to tell Dan how much I enjoyed our time together. I was quiet and shy, so it was completely out of my character to do that. But I just wanted him to know. I ran back into the hall, said just that, and left.

When I went back to Kettering at the end of that school year to finish my radiology degree, I asked my friend where her brother-in-law was. She honestly and seriously told me, "You don't want anything to do with him." But one year later, there I was, twenty-four years old, married to Dan, with a degree in MRI, living in Kettering. Dan had enlisted with the US Navy as I was finishing my schooling. I had only worked in X-ray at this point but was excited to start working in MRI. He was to be stationed in Norfolk, Virginia. New city, new life, new expectations, newly married. I was ready for change. The change I soon received, however, was not the change either of us expected.

Chapter 2

My First Seizure

Here we are, 1991. Dan and I enjoyed living in Hampton, Virginia, just on the other side of that amazing tunnel that goes underwater to Norfolk. We had only been living there for about three months, and I had not acquired a job yet. After settling into a little third-floor apartment, I started the dreadful job hunt. I handed out a few resumes, and called area clinics and hospitals, but things were just not happening. If a position came open, it would most likely be in X-ray. I could do that, but my heart was set on MRI. I loved it.

Then it happened. My first tonic-clonic seizure.

I always tell my doctors that my seizures started when I got married and question if there is any relation between the two (teehee).

Dan had no idea what was going on and although he hates for me to say this, he started CPR on me, as Dan mentioned in the preface. This shows you the general knowledge people had about seizure care thirty years ago. I believe we've moved forward with creating awareness in epilepsy, but we still have a long way to go. I am thankful for the progress made by all those seeking to increase awareness of seizures.

So, there was Dan, witnessing his first seizure. Poor guy, I love him so much. It scared him to death! Rightfully so. Those of us who suffer from seizures go through so much emotionally, but it is so important to note those people in our lives who witness them. What do *they* go through emotionally? Watching someone you love and care about have a seizure has got to be a painful and heart-wrenching emotional struggle no one can truly understand unless they go through it themselves.

Dan called 911. The paramedics had to take me on a gurney down two flights of very steep, very narrow steps. I wouldn't doubt for one second that part of that gurney hung over the balcony on the corners of that stairwell! I was obviously unconscious; otherwise, I would have totally freaked out and somehow jumped off that gurney.

Then came the usual. After the emergency room visit and CT scan of the brain, I had orders to follow up with a neurologist and have an MRI scan of my brain done. A little reminder here: We were new to the Hampton area, I had graduated with my degree in MRI, and I was previously searching for a job as an MRI technologist; to which I came up empty-handed. After seeing the neurologist, we made the appointment to have my MRI. I had performed so many MRIs, yet I had never had a scan of my own brain.

A little later, Dan took me to have an MRI of my brain. When the technologist called my name, Dan had to help me up and help me walk in because walking in a straight line was not an option for me. After the scan, Dan greeted us at the door and helped me gather my balance yet again.

The technologist was a very sweet lady, and we started talking. Dan mentioned that I had recently finished my MRI certification and I was looking for a job. Right away, I was embarrassed. Mind you, the technologist was helping hold me up because of the medication side effects, and I was using the wall for balance. Even so, she seemed interested. Seriously, she took my number and said she would call me because they were opening a new MRI unit at the Naval Hospital in Norfolk and were in search of skilled MRI technologists. *For real?* I thought. *I'm a mess, and she wants me to leave her my phone number?* So, no lie, about three months later, I got a call, and I got the job. Isn't it crazy how life works? God is so amazing!

Allergic Reaction to Medication

After that seizure, I was immediately put on Dilantin. As many of you know when starting a new medication, your body needs time to adjust. You are dizzy, nauseous, lethargic, have what appears to be non-ceasing headaches, and just all around feel like your head is a fishbowl half full of water with a vise grip being tightened on both sides. Just picture that for a second. Overall, however, I seemed to be tolerating the medication fairly well. Now isn't that last statement an oxymoron?

A few weeks before having that seizure, Dan and I had planned a trip to Florida to visit my family. When the time came, about a week after my seizure, off we went. I didn't look forward to the thirteen-hour trip to New Port Richey, Florida. We split the drive into two days, resting at a hotel halfway there. I was bored to death as a passenger the entire time. As you may know, I was not permitted to drive post-seizure. I had to be seizure-free for six months to be able to drive again. After what seemed like forever, we ended with our safe arrival in Florida and greeted the happy faces of my loving family.

That next morning, I started feeling very dizzy. I figured it was a normal side effect of my new medication, however, it kept getting worse. That night, it was so bad that I couldn't even sit up or turn my head without feeling like the house was running circles around me. I was helpless and without signs of improvement. Dan took me to the nearest ER. After what seemed like an eternity, as you know how ER visits can go, I was released with a prescription for Antivert for my dizziness. "That's it?" I thought. I mean this was some severe vertigo here. That night, Dan decided we should head back to Virginia in case anything worse happened. He drove all night nonstop as I tried to sleep, holding my head and not sure if closing my eyes helped mitigate the dizziness or leaving them open did. When we arrived home like two worn-out puppies that had run around all day, we both flopped on the bed and we were out.

I woke up earlier than Dan (a mystery of its own as Dan is always up before me), meandered to use the restroom, and totally freaked out when I saw myself in the mirror! I called out to Dan in a scared but not overly startling yelp (I didn't want to scare him). I swelled up twice my size and had a rash over my entire body, even between my fingers. Back to the ER, I went. I wasn't having any difficulty breathing, but the sheer look of me could cause someone else to stop breathing.

After several epinephrine injections without relief, I was admitted. I was soon diagnosed with an allergic reaction to Dilantin. Really? How many people have that kind of allergic reaction? Well, two to five people in every 10,000. I was hospitalized for a week, as it was quite an ordeal taking several days for the rash and swelling to start to subside.

The doctors and interns were excited though. This reaction was a medical-facility-swarming-with-interns dream. I have never seen so many doctors and interns in my life. Day after day, white coats headed to that second-floor hospital room to see the young lady with the Dilantin reaction. I am sure I was talked about for years to follow. I can just hear it now, "I remember when I was an intern at Portsmouth Naval Hospital when this young lady was admitted for an allergic reaction to Dilantin."

Due to the reaction, my doctors had to rule out Stevens-Johnson Syndrome (SJS), which can be a life-threatening condition. There are several causes of this syndrome, but most cases are due to an allergic reaction to a medication. There are several medications most likely to cause SJS. According to the Cleveland Clinic, the anti-epileptic drugs most likely to cause SJS are phenytoin (Dilantin), carbamazepine (Tegretol), lamotrigine (Lamictal), and phenobarbital (Luminal).[2]

As I read the other 3 medications included with possible SJS reactions in my recent research, I realized that I had tried them and they did not work for me! I suffered so much as my body rejected

---

[2] "Stevens-Johnson Syndrome," Cleveland Clinic, December 18, 2020, https://my.clevelandclinic.org/health/diseases/17656-stevens-johnson-syndrome.

each medication. I had no idea they were on the list with Dilantin. In my opinion, I should never have been put on those medications. This is a prime example of us needing to take an active part in our care.

To rule out SJS, I had to have an upper endoscopy done. This is when they stick a tube down your throat to take samples of tissue for testing.

I wanted to mention this because this story will always make me smile. As I am lying on the gurney getting ready, two good-looking young men are preparing everything for the exam. I was remembering a time when I was in X-ray school and working in the ER. A young man had just been given some pain medication and we wheeled him to our X-ray room to get pictures of his obviously dislocated shoulder. He was so medicated that he was telling us we had seduced him. We quickly corrected him by saying the nurses had sedated him to help with the pain. Once again, he said that we had seduced him. Sedated, not seduced, we chimed. I laughed inside.

Now, lying on the stretcher ready for my own procedure, I thought I would tell the guys my story about the young man and his dislocated shoulder. For some reason, the story got jumbled and as I was being sedated for the procedure, I remember telling them I was being seduced (just like the guy in my story). They quickly corrected me by telling me I was being sedated, to which I responded seduced. That is the last thing I remember before waking up in my hospital room again. Makes me laugh whenever I think about it.

A week later, the rash and swelling were subsiding, Stevens-Johnson Syndrome was ruled out, and I was released.

Adjustment Period

After some time adjusting, things started to get back to normal. One would like to think that things would go back to the way they were, but anyone with epilepsy knows that does not happen—at least not back to one hundred percent right away, and for some, never back to a full hundred percent. It takes time, and rightly so. Epilepsy is not an easy disease to deal with. Seizures are not easy to recuperate from. Memory is not easy to recover. Lives are not easy to reinstate.

Even so, I was able to start working again. Yes, that miracle job in MRI. God's timing is amazing! It took a little longer than expected, but soon, the MRI facility was open, and I began working. It was about four to five months after my first seizure, so Dan was my escort for about one or two months until I started to drive on my own once again.

When I started my first career as an MRI technologist, I worked hard to be the best that I could be. I took my career seriously. I tried to always go the extra mile. This didn't mean that I was any better than anyone else. I guess you can say that I was somewhat of an overachiever. I carried a little notebook to keep all my notes about MRI in. I would add to it daily. My husband reminded me that I was always willing to learn and share what I learned with other technologists. I loved my job.

In Denial, and Breakthrough Seizures

But as I tried to get my life back in order, I somehow tried to erase that diagnosis. Now, my denial was real. I insisted that I did not have epilepsy and I could come off the medication again and forever. Between the years 1991 and 2009, things were unpredictable. I would stay medicated for several years, just get so tired of taking the medications and dealing with all the side effects, and decide that I could start to come off the meds.

I in no way suggest this to anyone! This is a decision you need to make with your medical providers. I might last about one to two years before I would have another tonic-clonic seizure for an unknown reason. During this time, ninety-five percent of my seizures were occurring during the night (nocturnal) while I was sleeping. They would happen a few hours before I was to awaken. We had no idea what my triggers were, so I would instantly get back on my seizure medication. This on-off, on-off cycle went on for almost twenty years. It affected me in more ways than I can say: physically, emotionally, in my work, my intelligence level, my thought process, my self-esteem, my family, my husband, my … yes, my everything.

I have now been on consistent medication since 2009, 12 years now. During this time, I still suffered several breakthrough tonic-clonic seizures. What is a breakthrough seizure? I asked the same question. Why had I never even heard of this before? A breakthrough seizure is a seizure that has occurred after 12 months of being seizure-free and fully medicated. So it's like the medication appears to be working fine, then out of nowhere, bam! A seizure.

Just part of epilepsy, I guess. Just when you think things are going great, they suddenly don't go so great. No one will really understand the frustration unless it is you or someone you love having to go through the treatment process. There is no cure, just ways of dealing with it. So, we deal with it.

I am very happy to say that my last breakthrough seizure was 4 years ago. There is still controversy as to whether an aura is considered a seizure or not. I have heard some doctors say yes, it is a seizure, and some say no. It is said that an aura is actually part of a simple partial or focal seizure. Some define it as only a warning. There is some discrepancy here, therefore discussing this with your doctor is crucial. I had an aura yesterday, but it did not turn into a tonic-clonic seizure. With my doctor's approval, I am still able to drive and for me, we do not consider it a breakthrough seizure.

So, whether you are emptying trash bins for fifty cents a day, struggling to remember words and experiences, or changing your lifestyle to help avoid future seizures, stay tough. Anything free in this world anyone can get. It's the challenging circumstances and the fight of overcoming them that brings true success. God entrusts each of us with the joy of growth that comes from our trials, embracing them can be difficult, but the rewards far exceed the pain. What a beautiful thing to be able to stand tall and say *I fell apart, but I survived.*

Chapter 3
My Personal Seizure Triggers

So maybe you're bored reading about my past growing up. Does it really matter? Maybe. Maybe you were able to learn something through my story. I hope so. At any rate, please do not miss the points that are brought up in this chapter.

It has only been since 2009 that Dan and I have been attributing my seizures to specific triggers.

In 2009, Dan and I attended an epilepsy symposium at Vanderbilt in Nashville, TN. It was at this symposium that a doctor pointed out that continued AEDs could actually build up in the body and trigger a seizure. That was our scary takeaway.

It was around 2015 that we decided to go to an epilepsy symposium here in Asheville, North Carolina. Considering the ever-changing knowledge in the medical field, we figured we could certainly learn something. We did learn some things and got some small books that were helpful.

Although these educational events can be informative, what I want you the reader to understand, however, is that they could possibly be a little more intense than what you may anticipate. I will highlight my experience.

There were several classes to choose from, which made it kind of fun. In one meeting, doctors were scheduled to discuss different aspects of treatment for specific seizures. Pretty cool, I thought. I had a background in the medical field, so this would be informative.

The doctor was using PowerPoint and started to show a video of someone having a seizure. Right away, I was taken aback. To be honest, I was freaking out. I couldn't sit there. I couldn't watch, I couldn't listen, and I couldn't leave. It was like I was frozen in my seat.

Dan saw the distress on my face and quickly got me out of there. I was overcome with a heavy heart that completely overwhelmed me, and I just started crying in the hallway until I made my way to a room at the end of the hall. *How could I have subjected my husband to see me go through that? How could I not know what my husband had to see and what he had to deal with? How shallow of me!* Then I thought about how unfair epilepsy was! *Why did I have this disease?* Oh, then the flood of emotions started running over me! I cried a river.

This experience affected me for a while. It was too much for me at the time. Even now when I think about it, I get emotional. I'm sharing this because I want you to be prepared. Seeing something like that may affect you in ways you might not have otherwise considered. Maybe you want to see it, maybe you would rather exit the scene. Be prepared either way.

I completely understand that for those of you who are moms or dads with children with epilepsy, that type of information may be vital to the care you provide. God bless each and every one of you and your children! I cannot imagine.

Neither Dan nor I remember any classes in either symposium that mentioned neurotoxins and their effect on our brain, brain activity, and the possibility that they could trigger a seizure.

Reflex Epilepsies and Scent-triggered Seizures

As I searched and searched for documented statistics and information about smells triggering a seizure, I quickly realized that it is not common at all and extremely rarely reported. I discovered that seizures triggered by smells are called "olfactory stimulation" (smell stimulated). According to a recent study, olfactory function in epilepsy has not been thoroughly researched.[3] This is a new medical frontier! Scary and exciting at the same time! New discoveries have yet to be researched. I am already signed up!

After more recent research, I found out that I could have reflex epilepsy, or at least in part. There is somehow a link to smell and reflex epilepsies. I never knew to associate what I was smelling with my seizures until they started happening more frequently. My doctors never mentioned reflex epilepsies. This was truly an eye-opener for me.

What is Reflex Epilepsy?

Reflex epilepsies are a group of epilepsy syndromes in which a certain trigger or stimulus brings on seizures.

"The triggers in reflex epilepsies can be something simple in the environment such as movement or light, to something more complex such as reading or writing."[4] In my opinion, the triggers appear so random such as the sound of bells, listening to certain music, teeth brushing, or the sensation of being rubbed.

Have you heard of music being an actual seizure trigger? Or writing? Or drawing? I had not. Even though I did not see the word "smell" as a trigger to reflex epilepsy in a specific list, I did find an article verifying its rarity.

"Reflex epilepsies can be provoked by various types of external stimuli, but triggered by smell is rare..."[5]

Aha! So, smell-induced seizures are a part of reflex seizures; a very rare part. And, eighty-five percent of seizures of reflex

---

[3] "Stevens-Johnson Syndrome," Cleveland Clinic, https://my.clevelandclinic.org/health/diseases/17656-stevens-johnson-syndrome.

[4] "Facts about Seizures and Epilepsy," Epilepsy Foundation, https://www.epilepsy.com/learn/about-epilepsy-basics/facts-about-seizures-and-epilepsy.

[5] Faik Ilik and Ahmet Cemal Pazarli, "Reflex Epilepsy Triggered by Smell," https://doi.org/10.1177/1550059414533540.

epilepsies are generalized tonic-clonic seizures (grand mal). That is my most common seizure!

According to Wikipedia, reflex epilepsy is found in approximately five percent of people who have epilepsy. Photosensitive epilepsy is the most common type of reflex epilepsy, accounting for 75%–80% of cases.[6]

I am sure you have read about seizures triggered by photosensitivity; flickering lights, the sun shining off of objects, and the changing lights under a fan on the ceiling. Even though we have heard of them, they are not that common. Odd, I have always thought they were very common. It is suggested that photosensitive epilepsy occurs in about three percent of those diagnosed with epilepsy, giving it a rare tag.

Since there are such rare reports of smell-induced seizures, it seems only fair to assume it is less than three percent, giving it an even bigger tag of "rare" (less common than photosensitive epilepsy). There is not enough statistical data to delegate a percentage here. Is it fair to conclude that there are more people affected by smells than is suggested or reported? They may not even realize a smell is triggering a seizure.

Think about all the possible triggers for reflex epilepsies alone. Knowing about them now has made me more aware of my surroundings, more conscientious of epilepsy, and more sympathetic to those who are suffering more than myself.

As for me, I can say without a doubt, hands down, that certain smells have triggered a tonic-clonic seizure for me, and I have been able to document exactly what they are. Some smells I admit did not result in a tonic-clonic seizure, but other smells did. The smells that did not trigger a tonic-clonic seizure still had a negative effect on me neurologically and could have triggered a seizure had I not been medicated sufficiently. These smell-induced triggers include many icky odors. Friends and acquaintances I have

---

[6] "Reflex seizure," Wikipedia, https://en.wikipedia.org/wiki/Reflex_seizure#Epidemiology. Last accessed July 30, 2021.

chatted with through social media such as Twitter and Facebook have mentioned other smell-induced seizures due to the smell of hydrogen sulfide (rotten eggs), bad perfume, garbage, cleaning agents, a gas leak, a wet dog, pungent body odor, spoiled fish, and feces. As I went through the struggle of identifying my triggers, sharing my discoveries, and listening to others share their discoveries, I realized scent-triggered seizures are real, it wasn't just me, and it's something Dan and I feel passionately about sharing.

My Smell-Induced Seizures

Let's dig a little deeper as I explain the situations and smells that triggered a seizure for me.

Here I recall episodes in my life when I had a tonic-clonic seizure with a direct correlation to a smell that triggered it. Again, no one had even told us that seizures could be triggered by smells. This is something we figured out over the years by trial and error.

Repeatedly, Dan would sit down with me, once I was able to think again, and we would discuss possible triggers for that specific seizure. We would usually start with the most recent circumstance. He would ask me tons of questions until we reached common ground on the possible cause. As I have mentioned previously, we would talk about everything prior to the seizure. Where I was, what was going on around me, what had changed that would have normally been a part of that circumstance, were there other people nearby, were chemicals in the area, how long did I stay in certain areas, etc. We would slowly retrace in time, even to the prior day to get a full understanding of what the possible trigger could have been.

Here are some of the smells that triggered a tonic-clonic seizure for me.

2009

In 2009, I went to the kitchen to turn over some sweet potatoes we had cooking on a Teflon-coated hot plate on the counter. When

I walked out of the kitchen, I had a tonic-clonic seizure within one minute. When the seizure happens, as you know, we do not know it is happening. At least I don't. It takes some time, usually hours, for me to regain consciousness and start to think again. Soon after, Dan and I would begin our research. Why? Where? How? What could have caused it? Soon, we attributed this specific seizure to the smell of Teflon cooking. Back then, we were still a little unsure if that was the trigger. However, read the trigger in 2015 and you'll see why we feel confident in saying it was the Teflon.

2009

Later that same year, we were on a mission trip in Iquitos, Peru, and I had my hair cut at the local market. Not such a great idea in a third-world country unless you know about sanitary practices there. Boy, was I naive. Later that afternoon, my head was itching, and I felt like little crawly things were making their forever home on my head and in my hair. Oh great, I have lice. Thinking only that the little creatures must die, I went out, bought lice shampoo, and washed my hair that evening. That night, I had a tonic-clonic seizure. The estimated time between shampooing and the seizure was about six hours. We attributed that seizure to the lice shampoo.

2010

In 2010, I was getting ready to go to my clinical rotation for ultrasound. Yes. I was in school again. I just love learning, what can I say? Dan was out of town working during this seizure. We never really separated much, but this just happened to be one of those times. I seemed to be doing pretty well physically so off he went to a job in West Virginia. My mom lived right next door, so we decided he should take the job for the week. We had a beautiful dog named Cheyanne that had somehow contracted fleas. I went down to the lower level of our home to spray the area rug with flea spray. I figured since I was leaving for the day, it was a good time to let the spray set into the rug.

After spraying, I walked back up the stairs and felt that strong scary aura come on like a freight train. I said a quick prayer: *Oh God, please help me, please put your angels around my bed so I don't fall off.* I climbed on the bed, put a pillow under my head, and … and that's all I remember. I had a tonic-clonic seizure about one minute after smelling the flea spray. I am usually unconscious for one to two hours after a seizure. This time, I want to say about an hour later, I woke up. I do want to say that it would be safer to grab a pillow and stay on the floor rather than climb onto a bed.

It took me a minute to realize where I was and what had happened. I called my mom. She immediately left work. I want to say that that was one of the worst seizures I have ever had. I can't say for sure because no one witnessed it. The reason I say that, however, is because I had bruises all over my legs, bruises on my arms, bruises on my forehead, a bitten tongue, and busted blood vessels in my eyes. We of course attributed this tonic-clonic seizure to the flea spray.

2012

In 2012, one afternoon I was walking around beautiful Lake Junaluska, NC. They were repainting the shuffleboard a new shade of jade green. I could smell the paint as we passed by but seriously thought nothing of it. Soon after, I went home and lay down on a cot we had set up in the living room. (We had recently moved into our home in Waynesville, and our furniture had not arrived at the new house yet.) I had a slight headache and felt so tired. Dan was working on some things in the basement and heard odd banging on the floor above. When he came up, I was unconscious. I had had a tonic-clonic seizure. We attributed this seizure to the paint I had smelled earlier that day. I am estimating the time frame from smelling the paint to the time of the seizure to be about three hours.

2012

Another time in 2012, I was cleaning things up and doing a little decluttering in the kitchen. I came across a plastic container I had some half-used and almost empty pill bottles inside. These were bottles of vitamin B12, selenium, multivitamins, etc. I was checking the date on them to see if they could still be used. Some I just tossed in the trash and some I wondered if they were still OK because the date was fine. I opened a bottle of multivitamins—I can't remember the name of the brand—but I remember the smell was intense. Within one minute, I had a tonic-clonic seizure. We attributed this seizure to the toxicity of these specific vitamins. I do not know if they were outdated, and neither do I know the brand. I am sorry.

2014

In 2014, I had the opportunity to begin a new job. I was super excited because getting and maintaining a job when you are still struggling with seizures is quite a daunting task. I was hired as a part-time Spanish interpreter at the local Health Department. I was scheduled to work only two days a week for half a day. Great, I thought! Dan can drop me off and pick me up since it was only twice a week and only a few miles from our house. I once again was not allowed to drive yet, but this opportunity and arrangement were perfect!

The new local Health Department was a new building that was completely renovated out of an old Walmart store. On my very first day, I smelled something kind of odd but thought nothing of it. That night, I had a tonic-clonic seizure. We really didn't know what could have triggered that seizure, so we just let it go.

The following week, I went back to work for half a day. I smelled something odd in the air again. That night, I had another tonic-clonic seizure. Dan went back to see if he could smell anything. I swear Dan is the canary in the coal mine when I am not. We attributed those seizures to some type of sewer gas leakage.

2015

In 2015, we were over at a friend's house for dinner. Dan had agreed to help our friends fix one of their entrance doors as it was ill-fitted and the lock would not work correctly. Our friends were excited to make us some vegan-stuffed shells (which were amazing!). Yes, veganism can be very good. As my friend was frying the garlic, they accidentally got burnt a little. She lifted the pan to show me, and said, "Aww, man, Judi, look what I did!" I took one look, one small smell, and was overcome with a strong aura. I do not remember this, of course, but later they told me I looked scared, went to the door to go outside, but couldn't open it—it was the door the guys were fixing—went to the living room, lay on the floor, and had a tonic-clonic seizure. That all happened within ten seconds of smelling the burnt garlic. Once again, we asked all the potential identifying questions for possible triggers. This one was pretty straightforward tho. We attributed the seizure to Teflon burning once again. My friend was using a Teflon-coated frying pan.

2017

In 2017, we were working as ski instructors out in Colorado. I had a low back injury and herniated my disc at L2-L3 and was unable to teach that season. Man that was tough, being out in Colorado and unable to ski! I mean really! That was the entire reason we were there! I was still thankful though. Surrounded by majestic mountains and gorgeous snow. I was even given the opportunity to work part-time in the ticket center. That was actually pretty cool and I liked it. One afternoon, Dan and I decided we would enjoy one of the local hot spring spas not far from Summit County, Colorado. We reserved a private hot spring spa room. This was going to be a real treat. Sit down, relax, drink a cold cup of water, and enjoy each other's company as we relish in our own private little natural spring hot tub room.

When we entered, we could smell the sulfur, but it was natural, so we didn't think too much about it. The ground was stone and/or concrete. The room itself was like a big hollowed-out area of mountainside stone, with a bench on the side. Just beyond the bench was the hot tub, another area that appeared hollowed out of the stone wall itself. They had made two concrete steps with a side rail so you could step down into the hot tub, from where the steam was rising. We stepped down into the hot spring—oh, it felt so nice. Perfect temperature. We sat there and started to just relax.

Within about three minutes, I started to feel dizzy. Dan always takes control in even the slightest emergency, so when he said get out, I got out. Thankfully the bench was close and I lay down. Within about another minute, my hands and fingers started to freeze up on me. I had no control over the position of my fingers. They cramped up into an eagle's claw position, and I could not move them. I was so afraid and started freaking out and began to cry. What was happening? I thought I was having a stroke. I started to hyperventilate. Dan was Mr. Calm (God, I love that man). It didn't feel like the usual aura that would normally be my precursor alert to a seizure. I just felt that my body was reacting to something, and I had no control.

I do believe this was some type of seizure. Maybe not my normal tonic-clonic, but for sure some type of neurological response that I had never experienced before. Dan quickly opened the door trying to get some fresh air into the room. After a few minutes, I started to gain slight motion in my fingers. Dan acquired a wheelchair, helped me up, and got me outside to get some fresh air as quickly as he could. After about thirty minutes, I started to feel a little bit normal and was able to move my hands and fingers again. He helped me to the car, and we headed home. What an end to our sweet couples retreat spa day! We of course attributed that neurological response to the sulfur. There could be other toxins such as copper and zinc, but this particular hot spring was noted as having a stronger sulfur smell and content than the others. If we had only known. "Ambient sulfur dioxide (SO_2) is considered a risk factor for ischemic stroke and seizure, yet the mechanism of its effects on the brain is not currently readily understood."[7]

To summarize, here are my known, nearly 100% definite tonic-clonic seizure triggers:

- 2009 (twice): Teflon and lice shampoo

- 2010: Flea spray

- 2012 (twice): Paint and vitamins

- 2014: Sewer gas

- 2015: Teflon (again)

- 2017: Sulfur

Most of the triggers resulted in a tonic-clonic seizure. Sometimes within seconds, other times hours, or even the next day. With two of the triggers, I had to be exposed more than once, have another seizure, and then be able to pinpoint the cause. Most are without question, as they resulted in a seizure within seconds.

Often, I will experience other types of seizures such as absence seizures that we believe, once again, are triggered by smells and toxins. With many auras and seizures, we have not been able to identify the trigger. This is the case for most of my seizures and may be the case for yours as well. At any rate, these are examples of when smells once again were seizure triggers for me.

Significant Auras

An aura is a term that some people use to describe the warning they feel before consciousness is impaired, or before they have a

---

[7] Mieczysław Szyszkowicz, et al., "Sulfur Dioxide and Emergency Department Visits for Stroke and Seizure," *Hindawi*, March 18, 2012, https://doi.org/10.1155/2012/824724.

tonic-clonic seizure. An epilepsy aura is in fact **a focal aware seizure**. Focal aware seizures (FAS) are sometimes called warnings or auras because, for some people, a FAS develops into another type of seizure.[8] As I mentioned previously, there is still some discrepancy as to whether auras are considered seizures, but taking the above definition into consideration, I believe they are considered focal seizures.

Auras differ tremendously from person to person. Sometimes it's a feeling, a smell, a thought, or even a picture generated in the mind. I personally have a difficult time explaining my auras. I know what they are, and I prepare myself and my surroundings as it may develop into a full-blown tonic-clonic seizure.

Auras are a constant part of my life but often dissipate and do not result in a full-blown tonic-clonic seizure. I do want to mention four very, very significant strong auras I had that we believe were attributed to toxic smells.

2009

Dan and I were visiting friends in West Virginia. We were helping them work on a house and Dan was applying latex-based primer inside the home. I was helping with odd jobs inside the house. This was early on when we were still trying to attribute my auras and seizures to specific triggers. We had all the windows open and thought things would be okay. That evening, however, I had a very strong aura. We of course had medication on hand and quickly took some. We attributed this aura to the latex-based primer.

2018

In 2018, my husband and I were shopping at a large retail store. I had learned by now to be cautious of toxic areas, but I became a little complacent. I walked down the soap aisle as Dan went to the

---

[8] "Epilepsy auras," Epilepsy Society, https://epilepsysociety.org.uk/about-epilepsy/what-epilepsy/epilepsy-auras.

car to get something. Why on earth would I do that? Hello! Seconds later, I had a very strong aura, and I mean strong. I knew without a doubt I was going to have a seizure.

Let me pause there for a second and tell you something. During this time of my life, I was pretty low on faith. I believed in God but could not understand why God was allowing me to suffer. I kind of gave up, really, kind of had it with religion. But I tell you when that aura came in the middle of a store, I prayed, and I prayed hard. I said, *Lord, please stop this seizure! I know you can! Do not let this happen to me right here in front of all these people, please. I promise I will make it right; I will grow in my faith; I will follow you.*

Just then, a worker turned the corner of the aisle. I looked at her intently and told her I was going to have a seizure. I said please do not leave me, grabbed her by hand, and would not let go. She was trying to convince me to let go so she could go get help. Her pleas were not working. I sat down in the aisle, to a near lying-down position. I called Dan on my phone, texted him, and waited. Oh, it was coming, I was sure of it. I waited. I continued to sit there not letting this poor lady go. One minute turned into three, and three turned into five.

Dan came running down the aisle and put an Ativan in my mouth. Yes, I kept it in my purse but had left my purse in the car. Of all days! They brought me a wheelchair. Dan got me out of the store as quickly as possible to get me into the fresh air and then took me home. We attributed that aura and near tonic-clonic seizure to the numerous smells and neurotoxins in the soap aisle, which happens to be next door to the hair and makeup aisles. Toxins were galore.

You know, I totally believe that was a miracle. I believe God stopped it. That aura was so strong, there was no doubt in my mind that I was going to have a seizure. Yet, God proved His love for me at such a trying time in my life. I kept my promise; I grew in my faith and my relationship with Christ. Christ is a huge part of my life, even when I am weak. I am not perfect but growing in Him is a daily goal for me. He is amazing and has proven His love, grace, and mercy repeatedly. I thank Him over and over again. Even so, there have been times when my prayers to stop a seizure were not answered. I have learned to live with that and trust God anyway. Life is not perfect here on earth.

2019

Another aura was in April 2019, on my recent adventure at a ski area. I have never really had auras or difficulties when I'm outside skiing. So much good clean air in the mountains has always been healthy for me. But I will mention that I was skiing at a different ski area. My husband and I were waiting in the lift line when we both smelled something odd. My canary was concerned, but I was like, "Nah, I will be just fine, come on, we are outside!"

We made it to the top of the mountain, and as I skied off the chair lift, I had a very strong aura. I quickly clicked off my skis, threw my poles, sat down, and told my husband I was having an aura. Fortunately, right near us was a ski patrol building. Really? Thanks again, God! My friend Suzie went in and asked for a cup of water. I still think about it in amazement. Acres and acres of skiable terrain and I have an aura just steps away from the ski patrol building. Along with my cup of water came ski patrol to see if everything was OK. At this time, I was still having severe dizziness but that known, "going-to-have-a-seizure" aura was starting to fade.

They talked me into not skiing down, although I was adamant about waiting twenty minutes and skiing down a really cool blue mogul run! Could you just imagine skiing down a steep blue trail with moguls while having dizziness so bad it makes you walk like a drunken sailor? I admit that would have been bad. They took me down in the infamous red bucket. You know, that long red "sled" used by ski patrol to take injured skiers down the mountain. They strap you inside so you don't fall out. It has long bars in the front that the ski patroller holds as they ski you down in control. I will never forget that sweet lady ski patroller that took me down. She was an incredible skier as she controlled the bucket down some pretty steep slopes. I felt safe with her as well as the ski patroller that skied behind and beside me. I never thought I would ever have to do that, but there you go. I must say that ski patrollers are amazing! They took such good care of me and calmed my fears! God bless those wonderful people! I was doing well enough that, as we were in the middle of our descent, I pulled my phone out of my jacket pocket and filmed part of my trip down! Amazing views!

When we got to the bottom, my good friend Suzie was there at ski patrol waiting to give me my Ativan. That day was cut short. I am thankful for wonderful friends and ski patrol, well and of course my husband again. We attributed that aura and near tonic-clonic seizure to some type of oil used on the lifts. We of course could be wrong, but we both smelled it, and after the "post-seizure investigation" that my husband and I always do, the oiled lifts appeared to be the culprit. This is not normal for ski lifts. This happened to be a very old ski lift that had actually used old oil derricks to build the lift. With age, some burning of oil can happen unintentionally in the lift machinery. This is something I need to be very cautious and aware of from now on because of my love of skiing.

Since we are talking about skiing, I want to mention a friend of mine, Chuck. We used to work together in a ski area. He had been working as a snowmaker during the night shift and developed epilepsy in the last six to seven years. As his seizures became worse, doctors continued to increase medication doses, add new medications, and so on. Many of you can relate to this. His seizure activity began to affect his job.

Having to ride the lifts up and down the mountain started to become too dangerous. He told me that he started clipping himself to the chair lift using a carabiner. Really, dude, a carabiner? **This is not a suggestion to anyone that may be found in this or any similar "life-threatening" situation.** This is a story of a friend. Any type of work-related accommodations is between you, your doctors, and your employer. Chuck never knew when a seizure could possibly affect him, so he did what he thought was

45

the best choice at the time. When his seizures were not improving and getting worse and less predictable, he realized that snow-making was not the job for him. Because of his love of snowboarding, he has found another job at the ski area that does not take him thirty feet in the air alone at night.

2020

In 2020, I had an intense aura that I am sure once again would have turned into a seizure had I not been medicated adequately. We like to back our cars up near the front door of the house as it is easy to run out the door when pressed for time and just drive off. Normally, I walk to the side of the car if it's running, hold my breath, and put things in the back seat as needed. I can usually avoid any exhaust knowing we are outside with a lot of fresh country air. Unbeknownst to me, my husband was putting some things in the trunk and had left the trunk door open. I didn't even think about what I was doing and decided to just put things in the trunk as it was open and easily accessible.

Of course, the exhaust was right in my face. I held my breath as I always do but within two minutes, I was overcome with a very strong aura. I yelled for Dan, did the usual of lying down and grabbing a couch pillow to throw under my head, and told Dan I was going to have a seizure. He ran for Ativan and essential oils. My anti-seizure drug meds were doubled as I was coming off Vimpat and going on Lamictal at that time. Saved by meds. Just another environmental toxin to be aware of: exhaust. We no longer keep the car running when loading it.

Attributing Seizures to Toxins

The above-mentioned auras were strong enough that a tonic-clonic seizure was imminent. I just thank God they did not progress in that way. I will say that auras are a constant for me. I have them on average 1-2 times a week. Often, they scare me enough to stop what I am doing, grab some Ativan, grab a pillow to throw under my head, lie on the floor, and say a quick prayer. The intensity varies but I will always be ready in case a tonic-clonic seizure follows. I actually had one yesterday. I do not know the trigger, which is the case most of the time.

Of course, it took several years for us to be able to attribute my seizures to certain toxins. It also took several repetitive seizures before we were able to start to draw correlative conclusions as to their causes. Often, however, I have other types of seizures or neurological reactions such as twitching in my fingers, severe dizziness, lack of cognitive function, an odd thought process that I could not control, a time of uneasiness, a migraine, or something as simple as a headache. They are numerous and I am unable to mention them all.

The point here is that if I were not medicated to a therapeutic level, the auras could very well have resulted in a full-blown tonic-clonic seizure. The fact remains that even though I was medicated sufficiently to stop a tonic-clonic seizure, I still had an aura (also called a focal seizure) that was triggered by a neurotoxin.

Not every seizure or aura had a known trigger and oftentimes we were left still questioning the actual cause. However, I will include several possible triggers in Chapter 6. Please realize that toxins affect everyone in some way or another and can be manifested in completely different ways. This is a real issue we are faced with in our overly toxic world environment.

We believe that the medical field in general is so bombarded with this illness that it is easier to prescribe medication and treat the illness than it is to identify some of the possible causes. If we had not researched and continually reminded ourselves about the need to avoid neurotoxins in our life, what would my life be like today? I would have continued to walk down neurotoxic aisles in stores, breathe the fumes of burning Teflon, and all the while continue having seizure after seizure after seizure paralleled with increasing medication dosage.

Other Contributing Factors

Thus far, I have mentioned my personal triggers resulting in tonic-clonic seizures and auras resulting in varying neurological responses. I also want to mention other conditions that have been proven to affect me and my seizure activity. I am sure there are many contributing illnesses, but since I am only referencing those that have affected me personally, I will only name those.

Rheumatoid Arthritis (RA) and other Autoimmune Diseases

There is now a new classification of epilepsy called autoimmune epilepsy[9] which is caused by a change in immune function.

According to the Epilepsy Foundation: "We don't know exactly how often autoimmune epilepsy happens. It is estimated that 1 to 7 out of 20 (5%–35%) people with new onset seizures may have an autoimmune cause. These include people with a history of another autoimmune disease (such as rheumatoid arthritis, Graves' disease, Hashimoto's thyroiditis, Crohn's disease, ulcerative colitis, and systemic lupus erythematosus), a history of cancer, and a first-degree relative (parent, sibling, or child) with an autoimmune disease."

I was diagnosed with Rheumatoid Arthritis (RA) around 2005. Rheumatoid Arthritis, or RA, is an autoimmune and inflammatory disease, which means that your immune system attacks healthy cells in your body by mistake, causing inflammation (painful swelling) in the affected parts of the body. RA mainly attacks the joints, usually many joints at once. RA commonly affects joints in the hands, wrists, and knees. In a joint with RA, the lining of the joint becomes inflamed, causing damage to joint

---

[9] "Autoimmune Epilepsy," Epilepsy Foundation, https://www.epilepsy.com/learn/epilepsy-due-specific-causes/autoimmune-epilepsy.

tissue. This tissue damage can cause long-lasting or chronic pain, unsteadiness (lack of balance), and deformity (misshapenness).[10]

I can honestly say without a doubt that my seizure activity increased as I started having RA flare-ups. Coincidence? Maybe, but I doubt it.

I of course had no idea I had RA. I have no family history of it. I started having severe swelling and pain in my fingers, hands, wrists, shoulders, and hips. What in the world was going on? After several doctor visits, blood draws, and a plethora of other tests, I was finally diagnosed with RA. I would have intermittent flare-ups that were so painful there was no option except to take me to the ER. These flare-ups were so sporadic and so intense that any slight movement would cause excruciating pain.

A rheumatologist suggested I start taking the drug Methotrexate. Dan and I diligently researched the medicine, its side effects, and its uses. This medication is one of the most toxic drugs on the market and is used for treating cancer. Dan and I agreed: We needed to find an alternative means to battle my RA, so we decided I would not take Methotrexate.

What have we done about it? I drastically changed my diet and did my best to maintain an overall healthy lifestyle. Many of the changes I have made are dispersed within this book.

We were already vegetarians and eating fairly healthy, in our opinion. At this point, we decided to become vegan; still stay vegetarian, but now cut out dairy. The foods we eat play a much larger part in our overall health than many believe. I mean I wasn't giving the foods I consumed that much thought. We did some research about RA, foods to avoid, and foods to include in my diet. It became clear that eating a healthy vegan diet would only help. Avoiding saturated fats that are rich in cheese, butter, and meats was a must. The hardest part was omitting cheese from our diet. With time, it became easier, and now I don't even think about it.

---

[10] "Rheumatoid Arthritis (RA)," Centers for Disease Control and Prevention, https://www.cdc.gov/arthritis/basics/rheumatoid-arthritis.html.

We also became very aware of my sugar intake. We cut out white sugar altogether and only use maple syrup or raw cane sugar. With these changes in our diet, RA flare-ups became less frequent. When I did have them, they were not as severe and painful—well, they were still very painful, but somehow just a little easier to deal with. I still get them from time to time. Just last week, my right hand flared up. I was unable to hold things or use my hand very much at all for about four days. Since I learned that ibuprofen was a seizure trigger, I no longer take it.

Magnesium Deficiencies

There have been numerous studies about the relationship and role magnesium plays with those suffering from seizures. Some studies show lower magnesium levels in individuals with epilepsy as compared to those without epilepsy. There appears to be an overall consistency between the two, so I just choose to take magnesium supplements. Your choice, of course. I have no personal data about my intake of magnesium or how it has affected my seizures. I made such dramatic changes in my diet; it all kind of got lumped together. Check with your doctor about dosage if you decide to take supplements. There are several different types of magnesium as well. I mention magnesium and its importance in Chapter 8. The book I resource about epigenetics mentions this as well. Magnesium helps with bowel regularity and toxic constipation can also be a seizure trigger.

"Clinical and experimental investigations have shown that magnesium depletion causes a marked irritability of the nervous system, eventually resulting in epileptic seizures. Although magnesium deficiency as a cause of epilepsy is uncommon, its recognition and correction may prove life-saving."[11]

---

[11] D. Nuytten, et al., "Magnesium deficiency as a cause of acute intractable seizures," *Journal of Neurology*, vol. 238, 262–264, https://doi.org/10.1007/BF00319737.

Changing Hormones

Contraceptive management and seizure activity in women with epilepsy have been very complex and critical issues. There have been numerous studies showing increased seizure activity when taking oral contraceptives. Hormonal changes, correlative with a woman's menstrual cycle, are a well-known seizure trigger.

Here is my personal experience. About fifteen years ago, I had an intrauterine device (IUD) put in. Now Dan had already had a vasectomy, as getting pregnant was not an option for us as my seizures were not controlled and my medications were not "pregnancy friendly." Remember, this was thirty years ago. A lot has changed since then! I do believe pregnancy options while on AEDs have changed significantly and it is something you would need to discuss with your doctors.

After talking with my gynecologist, Dan and I decided that an IUD would help my menstrual cycles. I had very heavy cycles that lasted what seemed like forever, ten to twelve days, and were very painful. I was diagnosed with a bicornuate uterus which is shown to have a higher risk of miscarriages and preterm birth. Roughly one in every two hundred women has this congenital malformation. The uterus is shaped more like a heart instead of an oval egg (FYI, LOL).

Initially, the IUD appeared to be helping. About two months later, I started having pain in my lower pelvis. Of course, we always consider several possible reasons as we narrow down the possible cause. When the pain was getting more severe with sharp stabbing sensations, we decided to take the IUD out.

Please note, during the time I had the IUD in, I was having seizures more frequently. We already know that in some women, seizures can be more prevalent just prior to or during menstruation. Hormonal changes such as increased estrogen have been linked as triggers. Although IUDs do not increase estrogen levels but instead increase progesterone, the hormonal changes affected me and triggered more seizures.

I am not saying you need to have an IUD taken out if you have one. I am not saying that you should never have one. What I am saying is that, for me, there was a correlation between increased seizure activity while I had the IUD in. If this is something you may have concerns about, talk with your doctor.

I came across this great research article you may want to read, called "Do oral contraceptives increase epileptic seizures?"[12]

There has been a lot of discussion about IUDs and epilepsy. Hundreds of women have complained about increased seizure activity when using a Mirena IUD while other articles say it lessens the seizure activity in women. I know for me personally, it increased my seizure activity. Once again, we all respond differently.

Irritable Bowel Syndrome (IBS)/Constipation

There are studies stating that constipation can lead to a buildup of toxins in the system and may lead to an increase in seizure activity. But is there 100% proof? Not yet.

"The causal link between seizure and constipation is a common belief among patients and physicians, but there is no scientific data to support this association."[13]

But seriously, why is it common for me, and others that have mentioned this to me, to eliminate more feces than normal after a seizure? There has to be a direct correlation here. For me anyway, I was totally toxic. This toxicity triggered several of my seizures. I can say this with complete openness and honesty, as well as with a little embarrassment.

---

[12] Doodipala Samba Reddy, "Do oral contraceptives increase epileptic seizures?" *Expert Review of Neurotherapeutics*, vol. 17, issue 2, 129–134, https://doi.org/10.1080/14737175.2016.1243472.

[13] Leila Moezi, et al., "Constipation enhances the propensity to seizure in pentylenetetrazole-induced seizure models of mice," *Epilepsy & Behavior*, vo. 44, 200–2006, March 1, 2015, https://doi.org/10.1016/j.yebeh.2015.01.013.

Eating healthy and taking the time to care for your body and its elimination process is crucial. There is a direct correlation between the amount of exercise you get and the digestive system's process of elimination. Two peas in a pod, right? Diet and exercise. Eat prunes, and make sure you eat enough fiber. Well, I eat prunes anyway. I used to hate them, but now they are a fun snack. I exercise five to six days a week. Even if it's only fifteen to twenty minutes, I do it. Discipline my friends, discipline. On "bad" days, and you know what I mean, the last thing I want to do is exercise. I will force myself to do some yoga. Stretches really. I also try to take a short walk outside. Anything. The best time to take a walk is after a good rain. Seriously, there is cleanliness in the air after a rain because the air is saturated with negatively charged ions which purify the air of harmful substances. The fewer such ions in the air we breathe, the more tired we feel and the weaker our immunity.

I have changed my diet and eating habits in many ways. You will read more about that in Chapter 8. I try to eat at least a tablespoon of ground flaxseed a day. Flax seed has the nickname "flaxative." Due to my uncooperative digestive system, every little natural remedy can help. The magnesium citrate in the evenings has helped as well. I also will take aloe bitter sap from time to time. As the name suggests, these things are bitter! Water doesn't take the taste away so I down them with a glass of pure grape juice (no sugar). And then more water.

I will never forget one afternoon after my surgery; my sister was visiting with her girls. The middle girl, Jesse, age twelve at the time, was listening as we were talking about the crystals as I needed to take some. Anyway, she was like, "I'll take 'em." We laughed because we knew how nasty they tasted. I kind of feel bad about this, but I said OK, but we are going to chew them before we swallow them, I said. She was like "OK, let's do it" with a fun slightly cocky smirk on her face. As we each threw a couple in our mouth, I resisted the bite down as I heard her crunch her bitters with her teeth. Oh, my goodness, her face! We all started laughing to the point of crying as she was literally spitting it all out in the kitchen sink. I grabbed her some grape juice; my guilty feeling didn't pass as quickly as I had hoped. The lesson here; is don't chew them. Oh, and don't tell your niece to chew them either.

After a couple of days, if I am still unable to defecate, I will do an enema. Don't laugh, but I buy an enema bottle, pour out the chemical solution, and replace it with warm water and fresh lemon juice. I use the juice of one lemon with some warm water. It works and it is not full of toxic chemicals. All I can say is that I would rather do everything I possibly can naturally before putting any kind of chemical in my body. Honestly, this works.

Chapter 4
The Many Tolls of Epilepsy

Daily Thoughts from the Storm Front

Epilepsy is more than neurological storms in our brains that cause physical seizures. It's an emotional storm we deal with every day. And the days we are set back due to having a seizure? Well, that's a storm that can sometimes be bigger than life. It can cause depression, anxiety, pain, fear, and memory loss; cause us to question our self-esteem; and make us self-conscious, tired, and moody. It's not the fact that we have epilepsy that we may feel this way. I mean sure, that can be a little depressing, but it's more than that. Epilepsy is not a blanket diagnosis. What do we think?

If you don't have seizures, contemplate my almost daily thoughts numbered below. If you do have seizures, know that you are not alone.

1. When my brain has a storm, I can't think straight for hours after it.

2. This medication makes me feel dizzy, cloudy-headed, and just plain odd.

3. What if I have a seizure right in front of these people?

4. I just bit my tongue and can't talk right, can you tell?

5. Do I look as odd as I feel?

6. With my last seizure, I smacked my eyes and ended up with broken blood vessels. I must look horrible.

7. This medication is making my hair fall out, it's so ugly.

8. My head has been hurting most of the day. Will this ever end?

9. I'm so tired. I'm not lazy. I'm just tired.

10. Does that bright light bother you too?

11. I am so angry right now and I don't even know why.

12. Did I take my medication this morning? Oh no. I can't remember.

13. I must be such a burden to my family. I hate it.

14. I hate epilepsy.

15. I just want to die.

I could go on, but I won't. This swarm of emotions continually enveloping our minds is real. It's a daily fight. Is it just us? Is it our medications? Is it the illness? It seems that our anti-epileptic drugs (AEDs) have more side effects than there are minutes in a day. I will say from the very beginning, I do not like taking medications. Often, we have been quickly prescribed another medication to combat the side effects of the AEDs. Then, before you know it, you are taking four or five medications to combat the effects of the three to four other medications. In my opinion, take the minimal medications needed. I will be honest; yes, there are times when my emotions and depression are so out of whack that I just take it out on my husband. I go to him crying, saying I can't take this anymore, please help me get medication to help my depression. Somehow, through the grace of God, we make it through the tough times without adding more medication. We choose almost daily to preserve what health we can for our already immune-compromised mind and body.

The effects of seizures and their medications of course vary from person to person. **I am not going to say to anyone that they should stop or start taking certain medications.** That's absurd. This is between you and your neurologist and doctors. For those of you, like me, who cannot stop taking AEDs, let's see what we can do to help ourselves, as well as others. Anyone that suffers from epilepsy knows firsthand the struggles with emotions. I guess we may not be too far off from the general public on this point, yet there is a dimension only those with epilepsy can truly understand. I am sure you have questioned everything you are about to read yourself. You see, you are not alone.

Emotions and Faith

Merriam-Webster defines emotion as "(a) a conscious mental reaction (such as anger or fear) subjectively experienced as a strong feeling usually directed toward a specific object and typically accompanied by physiological and behavioral changes in the body, and (b) a state of feeling."[14]

Of course, you could add joy as an emotion, for example, so it's not just anger or fear.

But there you go. Our brain is the epicenter of mental reactions, feelings, and physiological, and behavioral changes. It seems to me that we cannot separate our epilepsy and the effects it has on our emotions.

Our compromised brain activity changes daily. Knowing that the many things we must deal with genuinely affect us is half the battle. The other half is to not let them control us. Yes, we are subject to riding the emotional rollercoaster, but we don't have to stay on the roller coaster all the time. Are there ways we can adapt and live a life where we can control our emotions a little more? I say yes. Read on.

Why?

I'm sorry you have epilepsy. I'm sorry that we live in a world full of sickness and pain. But take heart, our loving God is preparing a place for you in His kingdom where there will be no more pain, death, disease, crying, hurting, depression, or epilepsy! Amen!

You may be asking "Why do I have epilepsy?" I know I did, and still do sometimes.

---

[14] *Merriam-Webster.com Dictionary*, s.v. "emotion," last accessed July 30, 2021, https://www.merriam-webster.com/dictionary/emotion.

Epilepsy is not a punishment from God. In biblical times, it was believed that those who had seizures were being punished by God. They believed that satanic demons possessed them due to the individual's evil ways, and their seizures occurred when the demons were "active." Let me say this for sure: God is not punishing you. God loves you way too much! How could a loving God send demons into your body and watch you suffer? This thought process is not in harmony with the ways and principles of a loving God. Satan and the evil that exists in this world are simply a result of sin. When man fell in the Garden of Eden, sin started to invade the thoughts and practices of men. That same sin continues today. The devil, the originator of sin, *"roams the earth seeking whom he may devour"* (part of 1 Peter 5:8, NIV). God could have wiped Satan out with one word. But what would the angels think of a God like that? Surely, they would have obeyed God out of pure fear. That is not how God works. Sin will take its course while God proves His love by not forcing us to love Him back. It has and will always be a choice. We can choose sin, or we can choose Christ. Some things, we may not be able to wrap our heads around until we are face to face with Christ Himself, sitting at His feet, and hearing His loving answers. Have faith, just the size of a mustard seed, have faith. Let's not get caught up in the sin sickness, but instead, embrace the love that Christ poured out at the cross. Satan has already lost. God has already won. God is waiting patiently for each one of us to be a part of His kingdom. Let's focus on that!

So, your "why" could be attributed to many reasons. Maybe an accident you had, a result of drugs taken (prescribed or not), you may have a family history of epilepsy, you may have been born with it, or maybe your brain just overreacted to some unknown stimulus. Regardless of why you have epilepsy. Now, from here on out, we won't ask why, because honestly, there may not be a clear and definite reason. You as well as I just need to accept that there may not be an answer to why and move on.

Why Me?

You may be asking "why me?" Another possible unknown reason with no right answer that could possibly satisfy our personal need to know. One thing I will stand on for sure: God will never allow anything to happen to us that we will not be able to handle with His help. It may seem to you that you cannot handle having epilepsy, that you cannot deal with this sickness, and that God is not there to help. I was in that same dark tunnel of thinking. Sometimes, I still find myself walking toward that depressing tunnel from time to time, and I just have to stop walking. I have to get down on my knees and pray for help.

And we may even need help getting down on our knees. We have a loving God that hurts when we hurt and cries when we cry. Cast your burdens on Him, let Christ carry the load that we so selfishly think we can carry on our own. It's not something that we learn to do overnight, or even in a day or week. It's a lifestyle, a daily sacrifice of our will to that of His. Be encouraged. God has great plans for us. One of my favorite verses in the Bible is Jeremiah 29:11(NIV): *"For I know the plans I have for you," declares the Lord, "plans to prosper you and not to harm you, plans to give you hope and a future."* What a promise! Look to the future; be amazed at how God provides all that you need daily. The reasons why not-so-good things happen to us really cannot be answered. Job didn't know why he lost his land, his house, his family, and almost his life, but he remained faithful. If you have already lost faith, it's OK. We have all been called, and then called again. God will never give up on you!

You know, it is said that our trials make us stronger. Some are thankful to have such trials in their lives knowing that it may help someone else in some way or another. I am learning to consider it an honor to go through what I go through if it helps even just one person. Maybe it helps one person not have a seizure as I share what I have learned. Maybe it will help one person make a positive change in their life, their eating habits, their emotional struggles, their attitude, and their self-esteem. I don't have all the answers, but I do know that each one of us can be a blessing, a ray

59

of hope, a positive influence, a supporter, an advocate, or a rock for someone else. We need to accept that there may not be an answer to "why me?" and move on.

Wow, so far, we have no answers to "why?" or "why me?" Please do not think me unthoughtful or cold. I have thought and cried over these same seemingly unanswerable questions. I have decided not to question them anymore. What a burden lifted!

Depression

Depression affects more than fifteen million people or 6.7% in the US alone. It is real. It happens. It happens to others. It happens to us. This is something I fight intermittently, all the time. I know that sounds like an oxymoron, but I mean that it intermittently happens with consistency. When depression hits me, it hits me hard. It's like a dark cloud that hangs over me. It even feels heavy. It feels dark as it shadows my mind, crushes my body, and hangs on my face. I try to explain to my husband that I can't get out from under the clouds.

Maybe you have felt this. Maybe you feel it worse than I do. You are not alone and there is help. **Depression is not something that anyone should take lightly. Please seek help. Do not let it control you. There is help available. If you ever have thoughts of suicide, please call:**

National Suicide Prevention Lifeline

Hours: Available 24 hours.

Languages: English, Spanish.

800-273-8255

I know that I am very fortunate to have Dan. He has helped me through many bouts of depression as well as my darkest times when I felt that suicide was my best option. Bad episodes ended in verbal fights, which have left scars that have taken years to heal.

Good episodes ended with me beating on his chest bawling my eyes out until my body went limp from sheer exhaustion. I am thankful for him, and I am thankful for a God that loves me more than I can imagine! It's when these periods of deep depression ended on our knees is when our minds, bodies, and souls were lifted the highest.

Do What Makes you Happy

I believe one of the best antidotes to depression is doing something that makes you happy. Sounds simple, right? Maybe not so simple for some. A change of focus really. Instead of thinking about what you are unable to do, what can you do? You may still be able to do many of the things you enjoyed before epilepsy, with a few exceptions. Or, you may need to simply reduce the frequency and degree to which you do certain activities.

For example, for me, it's skiing. This is a sport that fills me up like none other. I swear there is snow running through my veins. Skiing is a huge part of my life. When my epilepsy started to poke its ugly nose into my ski life, it hit me hard. I didn't know how to handle the fact that skiing was not an option for me, for a time. Depending on the "stage" of my epilepsy—I know you know what I mean—sometimes good days, sometimes weeks of switching medications, sometimes a breakthrough seizure, and at other times, just life and the toll that seizures have on us in general, my skiing got put on hold. When my seizures were uncontrolled, skiing was not an option at all. Regulating our medications can be so arduous! Several times throughout my life, I couldn't even walk a straight line for at least six to nine months. My skiing life was affected, and as I said earlier, I took it hard. When I was able to get skis back on my feet, I wondered, *Why can't I ski like I used to? Why am I reacting slower? Turning slower?* I had to relearn everything every winter as a new season began. And it wasn't just my skiing, it affected my teaching of skiing as well.

It took time. That's the point I want to make here. With time, I was able to ski some mild green slopes (these are the easy ones, just above the bunny slope, for you non-skiers out there). For at least a year after a seizure, I would not go on a lift by myself for fear of having a seizure and falling off the lift. Even now, I don't like to ride the lifts alone. My skiing had to be dialed down quite a bit. Bye-bye crazy steeps, moguls, and beautiful white cornices. I was able with time to slowly increase my stamina and start skiing blue and even some mild black runs. Truth be told, the off-piste (off the trails), jumps, flips, terrain park, and crazy unheard-of speeds in the trees are what I really want to do but don't (dude, this is so difficult at times). I really can't take the chance of hurting myself or someone else.

But you know what? I am out in the snow, out in nature. I have skis on my feet, a helmet on my head, and goggles on my face (Thank you Idania for the coolest goggles ever). I am fortunate I am still able to do something that I enjoy so very much. I just had to dial it down a little.

So, think about how you can continue to do something that you enjoy, just dial down a little, a little less intensely, if you will.

Please note that if you are out west skiing at around 14,000 feet elevation, there is a huge difference in air availability! An even more reason to take it slow and allow time to adapt. It usually takes me two to three days for my head to stop spinning. Dan and I always acclimate a few days before we get on a chair lift. Even after that, however, I still feel light-headed and carry a little canister of oxygen on the slopes which really helps! As you may have figured out already, it's worth it for me. Not skiing is not an option if I can help it.

Doing something that you enjoy, something that brings you peace and happiness is a must. Slowly get back to doing something that puts you in your happy place. If your biggest pleasure in life has been completely blocked due to your epilepsy, I am sorry. An example could be playing football or ice hockey. These sports are so dangerous and not worth putting your brain in such a compromised situation. In these cases, you will have to think about something that may be a little less dangerous. This is something you can talk with your doctor about.

Wouldn't it be fun to try a bunch of different things to see which one takes you to your Zen place? Have you ever thought about skiing, biking, hiking, or tennis? How about other activities besides sports like painting, singing, learning a new language, playing an instrument, writing poetry, gardening, or cooking? Remember, getting back to some of these things you once enjoyed to the fullest may take time. Don't get discouraged. Take it slow, little by little. One step at a time still gets you on top of the mountain. It may just take a little longer. Playing the harp helped me after my brain surgery. I loved it! Unfortunately due to my RA, I had to let the harp go. I decided to forge forward with learning Portuguese. Why not? Work that brain muscle! I love it!

My Daily 3-step Routine to Help Battle Depression

Feel free to add it to your morning routine.

- **Smile**

When you wake up in the morning, smile. (It takes fewer muscles to smile than it does to frown.)

- **Gratitude**

After smiling, think of one thing you are thankful for and thank God for it. Just one. I had previously said three to five things, but when I was doing that, it seemed too quick. I have learned to focus on one item of thankfulness a day and take ten minutes to let it sink in as to how it affects me. Let me give you an example. One day, I woke up saying "I am thankful for my right big toe." Why? It gives me balance. When I ski, I lift up my right big toe to make a right-hand turn. Then I think of others that may not have a big toe. How has it compromised their life? Can they ski well? Do they limp? Can they dance? Does their right shoe have too much wiggle room making it uncomfortable? Does the skin around their ankles get irritated by the rubbing of an oversized shoe? Are they self-conscious when walking? Can they even wear flip-flops? If they do wear flip-flops, does the thong have to be moved over between the next two toes? I think this would irritate those toes because there isn't as much space as there is near the big toe. This would make the flip-flop lop-sided, with the pinky toe coming off the side at times. That would be so annoying. "Lord, I am thankful for my right big toe."

- **Sonder**

Live your day with "others-centered" love. Take the focus off yourself and reach a point of sonder.[15] Realize and appreciate there are others out there with equally complex lives and have compassion for them and for ourselves. This needs to be done daily. Make it a habit, but not mundane. Broaden your focus, and expand your thoughts. You are blessed.

Seizures in Public

No one can understand the specific emotion we feel about the possibility of having a seizure in public. It can be a daunting everyday emotion. What if I have one here, at the store, in school, or at the park? What if that little girl playing over there sees me having one? I could traumatize her life. What if I have one when walking down these stairs? Who will call 911? Could I have one while I am driving? What if I have one in a restaurant?

These scenarios are valid concerns. How do we know they are valid? Well, because they have happened to countless individuals with epilepsy. There is always that possibility. Therefore, there is always that emotion that comes with it: *fear.*

---

[15] Coined by John Koenig in *The Dictionary of Obscure Sorrows* (Simon & Schuster, 2021) and first written online at https://www.dictionaryofobscuresorrows.com/post/23536922667/sonder.

Know that you are not alone. I'm not going to tell you to just forget it or ignore your thoughts and move on. Instead, what I am saying is, to listen to your thoughts and take the necessary precautions. Be sure someone you are with knows you have epilepsy and what needs to be done if you have a seizure. If you are alone, I would advise having some type of identifier such as a medic bracelet. The bracelet gives me a little assurance and helps calm my fears when I am alone. Think about how your medication has stopped seizures in the past. Make sure you have specific medication with you such as Valium or the equivalent if it has been prescribed by your doctor for auras or breakthrough seizures. Make sure you have essential oils with you if you use them in addition to other seizure-prevention medications. I always keep my Ativan in the cute little oblong pill holder hooked to a key chain. The pill case is made for nitroglycerin tablets for people with heart conditions. My tiny little Ativan pills fit right in.

The point is not to focus on the fear of having a seizure. Here is an example. I love to ski the trees! The thrill of powder hitting me in the face and the challenge of skiing between beautiful evergreens is exhilarating! When teaching skiing, I tell my students not to look at the tree they may be skiing around. When they do, they have a higher chance of running right into it! It's true! I tell them to look between the trees. Pick your path and ski it. Focus on the task at hand, whatever it is you may be doing. Once you have redirected your focus, take a deep breath, say a quick prayer (I know it helps me), and enjoy yourself.

You are prepared, you are good to go. Don't allow yourself to stop living, or to continue living in fear. Don't dwell on what might happen. Don't look at the trees.

Self-esteem and Self-consciousness

I put these two emotions together as I feel they are very much related. Self-esteem refers to the feelings we have about ourselves (positive or negative). Being self-conscious refers to someone constantly questioning the way they appear to others. In my

65

opinion, one can drive the other. Think about it, if you are questioning if someone likes you and feel that they do not, your self-esteem may drop faster than a snowball melts in a bomb fire. Hey, it's ski season and my mind went straight to the snow. What can I say? But do they have to be connected? Can we have high self-esteem and still be self-conscious?

Why is it that we suffer so much from these two emotions? Is it our epileptic brains? Is it our medication? Is it just me? Is it just you? I don't think it's just me and I don't think it's just you. We cannot blame it all on our brains and I cannot blame it all on the medication. I am not sure why, to be honest. I feel some people handle these two emotions much better than others. There are way too many factors in our lives to make a clean-cut decision about why these emotions can tear us down. For some, it could be their childhood, their friendships, their lack of friendships, their marriage, their job, etc. For others, it's just who they are. But these emotions are changeable! Yes, we can change how we feel about ourselves. Yes, we can change how we think others feel about us!

I will say that my epilepsy has made me a very self-conscious person. Is that a true statement? Has my epilepsy made me this way? Or have I always had some self-conscious issues but have a real illness I can now pin it on? Well, for me, I think it is a little bit of both. My past has shown signs of insecurities and self-consciousness, but having epilepsy has, in my opinion, made them worse. I question everything. Not only once, but ten times on average. I decide, and then question that decision another ten times. I even question my question (is that possible?). With every inability to make a solid decision, I become more and more self-conscious and my self-esteem plummets. Then, there are days I kick it! Full of strength and vigor, ready to take on any challenge that comes my way! So much of it is simply our mindset. Where is your mind and what is it telling you? That you're weak and ill-fit? Or that you are strong and able?

There are so many ideas out there on the internet offering suggestions on ways to increase your self-esteem and learn to be less self-conscious. Here are a few of my favorite ways to strengthen me in these two areas.

Create a Growth Mindset

I really like what Dr. Carol Dweck of Stanford University had to say in one of her talks on "Developing a Growth Mindset." She is well-known for her research on mindset. In this particular presentation, she describes a high school in Chicago where, if a student did not pass a class, they would get the grade "not yet." She explains that if a student gets the grade "not yet," they are on a learning curve, giving them a path into the future. It gives them a growth mindset proposing that talents, strategy, resilience, and self-esteem can be developed. Such a contrast to a failing grade which gives the idea of a fixed mindset without room to grow.

Add "not yet" to things in your life that you are still working on. Give yourself an opportunity.

Have I learned the harp well? Not yet.

Have I lost the weight I need to lose? Not yet.

Can I speak Portuguese fluently? Not yet.

Can you walk a straight line? Not yet.

Can you drive? Not yet.

You are a beautiful work in progress!

Engage your Body, Mind, and Soul with a Good Diet, Exercise, and Rest

I know that when my body is feeling healthy, I'm eating well, and I can maintain some type of exercise, I do not get as depressed. I feel better about myself and get more done that day. I know that exercise is not always possible. I have those days too. During those times I make myself do stretches, yoga, and maybe a little upper

67

body weight training. I do not do anything that messes with my already compromised brain. For example, I do not jump up and down, move my body up and down, or turn my head quickly from side to side, no squats, nothing that puts my head below my chest, and no burpees (I'm so sad, lol). I do the best I can on bad days to keep my body in shape. Feelings of inadequacy can grow when our body is weak and tired, and if we are moody and negative. It is difficult to slow the mind down and replace unhelpful thinking patterns when the body is restless, exhausted, or malnourished in any way.

Live your Life

Do what brings you joy. Who cares what other people think? They have their lives. You have yours. Shrug your shoulders and do your thing. Don't give other people that much power over your life. Do things. Do things you never thought about doing before. I mean why not? The more you get out of your comfort zone, the more you'll understand that you don't need to let low self-esteem or self-consciousness hold you back. This sounds like so much fun already!

"Never bend your head. Always hold it high. Look the world straight in the face." —*Helen Keller*

Hey, you are amazing! Anyone that suffers from seizures struggles with depression, and wonders how to just live another day, I praise you for not giving up. Epilepsy is not a medical condition that people understand and easily accept. Medicine still does not know what triggers our seizures, how to stop them, or how to cure us. This doesn't make you a victim of epilepsy. In a way, maybe it should empower you. How can I, and how can you make a difference? There are over 3.4 million people with epilepsy in the US alone. Here is where you must find what works for you. Maybe join an epilepsy awareness Facebook page and be a part of something greater than yourself. Comment with words of encouragement. I think we all could add more success stories on these Facebook pages anyway. Let others know what good things you do for others (you're not tooting your own horn, but you're being open as others may like your idea and do it as well). Let others know how they can be strengthened and how they can strengthen others. Join the Epilepsy Foundation on the internet as there is so much to be gained as we band together searching not only for a cure but ways to minimize the effects of epilepsy and learn how to deal with and avoid certain triggers. Low self-esteem and self-consciousness are temporary. Don't let them set up camp in your life. You have the final decision here.

Dealing with Stigma

I mentioned stigma in the beginning. I do believe it still exists, but what do we do about it? I have a very hard time fully understanding if people are really treating me differently due to my epilepsy or if it's just my imagination.

Maybe we are treated a little differently, and at times it is a blessing and very much needed. Don't get me wrong, even though we do not want to be singled out, sometimes, we may need a little more "understanding" and this can go a long way when given by people who understand, care, and love us.

Now, when it comes to feeling like others may treat you differently, in a negative way, maybe just try to feel loved. I mean we can't let this control us. Most people will never know that you even have epilepsy. But what about the outward signs? Our dizziness? Our "brain fog"? Our lack of self-esteem? Our "differentness"? Some of us do fight the battle of stigma. No matter how hard we try to be and do things just like everybody else, sometimes, we just can't. Well, that's awesome! Who wants to be like everybody else anyway? Maybe there are things that may limit you in one way or another. For example, I cannot walk down the soap aisle in a department store. I cannot ski that double black off-piste run that I used to ski. Maybe you cannot get in a hot tub with friends or cannot watch a movie that has seizure-triggering computer animations. This is understandable. And for those that see you as "odd" or "weird," well, that is their loss. What a privilege to know someone that fights the battle of epilepsy every day! I say embrace it and hold on to God's love, and you win!

The most productive path for breaking the stigma attached to epilepsy is spreading awareness and increasing knowledge. Not just increasing our knowledge, but everyone else's. Much of fear comes from the unknown. People that do not know about epilepsy are, in a sense, afraid. Maybe just afraid of something they do not understand or know about. Coping with fear? Well, that's different for everyone. Some people can become mean, exclusive, judgmental, and just plain hurtful. Sometimes, people can treat others differently through ignorance. They honestly do not know how to act. Our ability as supporters of epilepsy awareness is to break the stigma. We are sharing our stories, sharing our trials, and sharing our triumphs.

Support Groups

Support groups can be such an encouraging resource. There are many support groups out there. Find the one that works best for you. There are national groups, state groups, local groups, Facebook groups, etc. Here are some options.

1. Epilepsy Foundation: https://www.epilepsy.com (national, state, local groups)
2. My Epilepsy Team: www.myepilepsyteam.com
3. Some Facebook Groups:
   a. @epilepsysupports
   b. @EpilepsyFoundationofAmerica
   c. @EpilepsySupportGroup
   d. @EndEpilepsy
   e. @EpilepsySupport
   f. @TeamEpilepsy

*and several other possible Facebook groups

4. Twitter has been a wonderful resource for support, sharing, and learning.

Hang out and consider joining the one that fits best for you. We are all different, and the groups are different as well.

Friends

I have heard heart-wrenching stories of friends that quit being friends when they found out that they had epilepsy or boyfriends/girlfriends that broke up for this same reason. Really? Are they that shallow? Who wants friends like that anyway?

As I stated before, you are a privilege to know. You are a blessing to be around. You fight daily and they have no idea! You are stronger than so many people! You are an inspiration! Wow! You are amazing! The power you have is nothing to scoff at, nothing to be made fun of, and nothing to take lightly! Who cares that as we laugh with friends reminiscing, sometimes we can't remember a thing about what we are laughing at?! Laugh anyway. I do, and as I am laughing, I am saying that I have no idea what they are talking about. Then, we all laugh even harder.

There is an old saying: "Good friends are like stars. You don't always see them, but you know they are always there." Be the friend you would want to hang out with.

Workplace

Friends and family are one thing, work is another. I am simply going to mention one thing about work and move on.

If you are lucky, work may be interrupted for a short amount of time and then you are able to start back up again. That was my case and I feel very fortunate. For others, changing jobs or even ending a job may be the only option for them. In this case, it's easy for me to say "cool, try something new." However, if I couldn't teach skiing anymore, I would be devastated. Personally, I say don't throw the baby out with the bathwater. Working part-time may be a wonderful option for you. Maybe starting a new career could be exactly what you need. No matter the avenue here, don't give up. Life can be so exciting when new opportunities present themselves. And, we take them.

"In the United States, the Americans with Disabilities Act makes it illegal to deny someone a job because of a medical condition if they can perform the essential duties of that job. People who feel they are being discriminated against because they have epilepsy should consider seeing a lawyer who understands disability law."[16]

Finances and Economics

I feel that having seizures affects everyone in some way or another economically. Maybe it's because working a regular eight-hour-a-day job is not possible for you. Maybe you care for a loved one and miss out on work yourself. For many, it's purely the inability to drive. For me, the repercussions were substantial.

Jobs

Before my epilepsy got out of control about fifteen years ago, I was bringing in the regular bi-monthly paychecks as well as my husband's. My job in MRI was lucrative. I enjoyed it. Bills were paid on time, extra money for eating out was available, and a splurge here and there to the movies was totally doable. When this was interrupted, our finances hit a brick wall. I know we are all taught to put money aside for emergencies. Well, that money aside just didn't cut it. Although my husband was working in construction, he could not make it to work on a regular basis. He lost work every day he cared for me, which was significant. He was unable to leave me alone. As doctor appointments were made, he

---

[16] "Social Concerns," Epilepsy Foundation,
   https://www.epilepsy.com/learn/challenges-epilepsy/social-concerns.

missed work. As more diagnostic tests were needed, he missed work.

I am sure that many of you have lost your jobs due to the inability to consistently just arrive at the job site. Many spouses have lost their jobs as they became caregivers. I couldn't drive for three years, so Dan had to take me everywhere. Even to my yearly woman's appointment. Poor guy, sitting in the lobby with a handful of women glancing at him wondering, "What in the world is he doing here? Poor fella."

As we struggled to stay afloat financially and my seizures continued, being unable to pay things on time, we got a little behind. This was not the norm for us.

Mortgage

Mind you, we were living in a beautiful home we had built. I had designed it and we had built it together. Angled kitchen, large A-frame living room with cathedral ceilings, all glass in the front to bring in the sun and mountain views. Spiral staircase to the basement where the pool table was. Tongue-and-groove wood on every wall. It was a cabin in the mountains of Western North Carolina, right up against the Great Smoky Mountains. Honestly, it was not a huge extravagant home, it was small, maybe 1,300 square feet. But it was ours. We built it with a labor of love.

As the bills kept coming in, we were unable to continue to pay our mortgage. I had always wondered if the police actually come to your door when a home is about to go into foreclosure. Well, they do. I was overcome with guilt. Because of me, we were going to lose the house that we put our money and sweat equity into building. I loved my home. Seeing through the dark tunnel, we continued praying that God would take care of us, provide for us, and lead us through. We started putting up ads, for-sale-by-owner signs, etc. If we could just sell it, that would be a miracle. No lie, about two weeks before the bank was about to rip it out of our hands, we had a buyer. Seriously. We closed within two weeks. We did not lose any money, and we did not owe any money, but we didn't make any money either. That's OK. I'll take it. A foreclosure would have hurt us far worse.

Even though I think of that home from time to time, a little sad, I thank God we were able to sell it. God knew. We just needed to trust in Him. The huge learning curve here: when you are losing your home, and cannot make the full mortgage payments each month, make part of it. Pay as much as you can. When I called the bank in desperation, they told me to just stop paying. I was like "don't pay anything?" The bank responded, "Nope, don't pay anything." I was so naive! They saw the pictures of our home. They knew it was worth more. They knew they could sell it. The thought makes me sick. I feel so cheated by the bank. That was just plain wrong of them. Oh well, Judi, let it go.

Rings

At some point in all this economic trial, we took our wedding rings to one of the local "We Buy Gold" stores. Never thought I would ever have to do that. We discussed it, we loved each other enough to know that the rings were not what our marriage was about. Besides, I had so much swelling in my fingers due to rheumatoid arthritis and acromegaly (which I did not yet know I had) I wasn't even wearing mine. Yes, they meant something to us. No, it wasn't easy. Sometimes you just gotta do what ya gotta do.

I don't have all the answers, but looking back, I do wish I had been more frugal. More aware, making provisions for hard times, and downsizing. Little things that may have helped us in a big way, well, we really didn't think about them. Here are some things that may help you prepare for times that may be a little harder. If you are unable to drive, ask friends and family to take you to appointments so your spouse doesn't have to miss work. Sell the things that you do not need. Go over your budget and save wherever possible! Less travel and gas, less eating out, less binge buying. Buy your groceries at discount stores; use Amazon if it works for you. When physically shopping in stores, it is more likely that you will buy things you do not need. When ordering online, your purchasing is much more intentional and less "spur-of-the-moment buying." I wish I did more online shopping back in the day. It was not as common as it is now. You have it better already!

Disability

Many of you may be trying to apply for disability. When my seizures became more frequent and uncontrollable, we started this process. It took a couple of years and a couple of denials. I finally hired a lawyer, and it still took a couple of years more. I finally was approved. Don't give up. It may be difficult to get approved, but many of us need that check to make ends meet. I do suggest hiring a lawyer. Without a lawyer, I do not think I would have been able to successfully receive disability. My social security check was a huge blessing for us as we started the long process of getting out of the debt we had incurred.

It took time for us to build our severely damaged credit back up again. Believe it or not, we are still dealing with fixing our credit. And it has been about fifteen years! Slow and steady. We are blessed, and we are thankful. Dan has been able to work more over the last few years, and we continue to teach skiing when we can. I'll just focus on that. Oh, I may not have mentioned this earlier, but Dan teaches skiing also. We go together, and that helps me feel even more confident when I am out in the snow. Just knowing he is somewhere on the mountain not too far away helps calm my soul. I do hope that with time, I feel confident enough to head out on the mountain alone. (Side note, lol)

I do feel there is a stigma with receiving disability benefits. It has made me very self-conscious. I feel embarrassed when going to a doctor's appointment and showing my Medicare card. They ask, why do you have Medicare? You are not sixty-five. Are you on disability? One day, I cringed when a neighbor was standing near me at a doctor's office as I was checking out. Really? You have the same doctor as me, and you just happened to have an appointment at the same time as me? What are the chances? I was so embarrassed. I had to get over it. I had to remember all that I had been through and that people have no idea. We cannot worry about what others think. They are going to think what they want to think anyway. I can't let issues like this bother me. And you shouldn't either. My new mantra is "Learning not to care what people think, without stopping to care about people."

Driving

Not only do we get prescribed medication that makes us feel like we are emotionally on trial, but we also get our driver's license taken away for a period after a seizure. Bye-bye independence!

Now, depending on your state, the rules are different. Here in North Carolina, you must be seizure-free for six months in order to start driving again. As I mentioned earlier, I lost mine for three years. I lost it again for three months sometime after that due to a medication change. And again, three months after that during another medication change. As with so many trials that epilepsy brings, we and our partners learn to deal with them.

I remember a time when things were going fairly well. My medication was keeping my seizures at bay, but I was not even close to the 6-month "get my license back" deadline yet. I was so antsy to get a little independence back that Dan and I decided we could buy a moped. Perfect I thought! I was totally game. Even though we lived in a rural setting, we only lived about 7 miles from the nearest grocery. I would tighten my helmet, velcro my gloves, and hit the road. It felt amazing! I just loved it! I would park in front of the grocery and walk in by myself. By myself. Shop a little by myself. I used essential oils like lavender to help with smells and breathed through my mouth the entire time in the market. I avoided the soap isles, and made my visit quick, but, it was so nice! When I was able to get my license back, I sold the moped.

Something I never knew...there may be a little stigma with a moped. LOL. Some individuals that use them regularly have had their licenses taken away due to drinking and driving. For them, it's called a "liquorcycle." I laughed so hard. Well, call it what you like, but for me, it was a breath of fresh air!

The Department of Motor Vehicles (DMV)

I'll never forget sitting in the lobby of the DMV. I had to renew my license (yes, Dan drove me and was waiting patiently outside). I had never told the DMV of my condition. I never had to, or so I thought. I knew the rules. I never drove without waiting the required six months. I can say that with sincere honesty. At this time, I was not driving, I just had to renew my license. But there I was, about to see my red number show up on the screen just above the doorway. I was a little nervous thinking this whole seizure thing could really mess things up. Finally, my number blinked red and I headed to the desk in the back where this sweet-looking lady was seated. No worries so far.

"Here is my old license, I just need to renew it," I stuttered. I'm thinking, take the eye exam, and bam, I'm outta here. Then the questions about my medical history and if I had any condition that could possibly be linked to affecting my ability to drive began. Then the final deadbolt question: "Do you have seizures or epilepsy?"

I wanted to say no so badly. All the while I was thinking, "Please don't take my license, please don't take my license." But I said yes, I have epilepsy. And that's it. I walked out without a new license. Yes, I cried.

Let the paperwork begin. I am now in the DMV computer system as having epilepsy and am placed on the "medical advisory" list. This is how it worked for me here in North Carolina. The state sent me a form that I had to take to my doctor to verify when I had my last seizure. I then sent that paper to the DMV, and they kept track of the timeline. Once the six-month seizure-free period had passed, they sent another form to verify that I had been seizure-free for six months and I took it to be signed by my doctor. We had to repeat this last process several times as it took a while to keep my seizures at bay for six months straight. Finally, my doctor signed it, I mailed it, and I was taken off the "medical advisory" list. When this happens, you get to head back over to get that precious little plastic card with your "not so cute" little picture on it. What a great feeling.

Telling the truth about having seizures was hard. But think about it for just a moment. If you lie, and then actually have a seizure when driving? What if someone was injured when you had this seizure? Or worse, what if someone was killed due to your lie? I know that I would not want that responsibility or guilt on my shoulders. Go through the more difficult process of staying legitimate. It's totally worth it. Everything has its time and season. There are reasons life happens in the timeframe it happens.

At any rate, I found a great link on the Epilepsy Foundation website[17] that lets you put in your state so you can see the rules. You can also check with your local DMV.

Making Provisions

Making provisions for your life, in general, may indeed help you as it did me. Here are some things to consider.

- **Online Shopping**

Try to do all your shopping online if you can. As I mentioned earlier, Amazon Prime is a terrific option, although I dropped Prime not too long ago, as paying the yearly fee was a commodity I could let go of. If you order $25 or more with Amazon, you get free shipping. Yes, the packages may take longer, a week to ten days on average, but hey, it's free. I love it, and you only need to walk out the door to pick up your package on the doorstep.

Walmart also offers a pickup option as well as free delivery on orders $35 or more (this may vary). You could order what you need and ask a friend or family member to pick it up for you. This is easier for them, and they are more willing to do this than shop for you.

---

[17] "State Driving Laws Database," Epilepsy Foundation, https://www.epilepsy.com/driving-laws.

Lately, with COVID-19, stores have stepped up to the plate in a huge way. I now do all my grocery shopping online, drive to the pick-up parking area, pop the trunk, and the attendants put everything in my vehicle. Prices vary for the commodity. Aldi charges $1.99 and Publix is free. These charges vary, I am sure. This is a wonderful service! I wish they had done this before this pandemic!

- **Plan Ahead**

Schedule things ahead of time and set up family or friends to take you. I know, I know, this can be so degrading and difficult. It was for me. What makes it even harder is when a friend tells you, "If you ever need a ride, you just let me know." And then when you drum up enough nerve to ask them, they are like "oh, uh, I really can't..." Don't let this discourage you.

Preparing and scheduling ahead of time is vital. Remember that being in a car with someone who uses a strong cologne or perfume could be a possible trigger (they are for me). Those little car-smelly things people put in the vents are just as bad. Ask your friend not to use them. They will not be offended if they care. Also, a new car has very strong smells such as benzene so be aware of this as well as other smells that could possibly be a trigger. Another reason I carry lavender oil and keep the vehicle windows down.

- **Carpool**

Find out who lives close to you and set up carpooling. Coworkers are usually pretty good about this, but keep in mind you will need to keep up on this at least on a weekly basis, or at least until it becomes a set procedure, so no one forgets. I forgot to confirm a friend was picking me up one morning. After about thirty minutes, I called my friend and calmly eased into the question, "Where are you?!" She turned around and headed right over.

Let coworkers and friends know that you appreciate them. I did this just this past month. I had been seizure-free for about three years! Yay! Then, I had two seizures in two months. I am now back to relying on others to take me places. Anyway, surprise them from time to time with a gift. Good friends usually do not want to take your money. I gave my friend some essential oil-infused dark chocolate candies from doTERRA the other week. She enjoyed and appreciated them so much. It made me feel good too.

Driving on Your Own Again

Once you start driving again, I recommend not driving alone for a while. I don't know, I just felt better knowing that someone was there in case I felt weird or something. I was overly cautious and kind of weird about it. I would look both ways before starting out into an intersection like three times. When changing lanes on highways, I would do the same thing. It took a little while for me to relax and still be cautious. Once I started to feel comfortable behind the wheel and wasn't afraid of a seizure, I started to drive short distances alone.

Now, something to consider and be conscious about is pumping gas. I do not pump my own gas. Whenever our vehicle needs gas, my husband refills it; even if that means just driving down the road to fill it up and coming right back home again. My friend saw Dan driving away to put gas in the car and she was like "Really? Why doesn't my husband do that?" In this case, being treated a little differently is cool. For me, gas is a seizure trigger. It may not be a known trigger for you, but just be aware that it could potentially be one.

When my husband and I are driving somewhere, and we need gas, he always pumps it while all the windows are up so the fumes do not enter the car. Sometimes this is difficult, but we do the best we can. On very hot days and very cold days, I wonder why all the pumps are on sloth time. "Hurry up, the temp in here is starting to freak me out." I still breathe through my mouth until we drive away and can put the windows down and get some fresh air. Stay away from gas fumes if possible. If I am with my husband and I must run into the store to take a quick bathroom break, I breathe through my mouth the entire time. This has been such a norm for me, I don't even realize I am doing it anymore. Since the COVID-19 pandemic has required mask-wearing, things have been easier for me. I actually appreciate the masks and how they have helped me avoid strong smells and neurotoxins.

Short and Long-term Memory Loss

Seizures have a direct link to memory loss, both long-term and short-term memory. I realize this is nothing new for many of you reading this, but when it gets worse and worse with time, it starts to really take its toll. It's not just the seizures, mind you. Our medications affect our memory, both long-term and short-term as well.

Great, now what, right? Well, lucky for you (and me), our brains are considered to have a high rate of plasticity. What exactly does that mean? Well, basically, the brain is a muscle. Muscles get weak, but they can also get strong again. So, work that muscle!

Activities to Strengthen Your Memory

Do you know what I am doing? I am learning the harp. Yup, over fifty years old (yup, the secret is out) and I am learning to play the harp. Not only is it strengthening my brain, but it is also so calming to my soul. Let me tell you though, it's hard. Not impossible, but it for sure takes dedication and perseverance! I also love to do crossword puzzles. I am in no way as good as my mom, as the easy ones can be a challenge for me to remember words, but I do them anyway.

I also like to read good books. Spending too much time on the computer is not good for us anyway. Grab a book instead. I have a few favorites such as the books written by Ellen G. White, "The Desire of Ages" (my all-time favorite), and "The Great Controversy." I love any book about World War II based on true stories of people that struggled, called on God, and made it through insurmountable difficulties, such as the book "Flee the Captor" by

Herbert Ford and "A Thousand Shall Fall" by Susi Mundy. I love books about motivation and positive change in your life such as "The Obstacle is the Way" by Ryan Holiday and "Hard Optimism" by Price Pritchett. I am now reading (listening to, actually) "Girl Wash Your Face" and "Girl Stop Apologizing," both by Rachel Hollis.

(Although, on a side note, I am bummed that Hollis and her husband are breaking up. Aren't her books about perseverance? Making life work? Giving it your all? I am saddened that they called it quits. Yet, we never know the whole story. I am in no way passing judgment. I am just a firm believer that all things are possible through Christ. Marriage is no different. It does take two, but I know God gives even one enough courage and strength to make it work. I know He did for Dan. My emotional state caused me to give up on my marriage too many times. Dan was strong and I thank God for that.)

There are many more books out there worth reading. Don't waste your time on fiction, fantasy, and romance novels. Real life is where it's at. Dan and I often read a book together, a chapter a night. It is something that has bonded us in a special way. The last book we read together was "Unbroken" by Laura Hillenbrand. Wow, incredible story!

My point here is the need to exercise your mind. Read, learn a new language, play a new instrument, pick a new sport to play, put a puzzle together, or start doing crossword puzzles, anything that makes you think—anything that can exercise that most important muscle in our body, the brain. Look up these books, and order the book or the audiobook. I do not order e-books. I feel the time I spend on the computer is too much already. I look at reading as a break from the computer. If possible, read the real print. If it is a new book, I do let it air out a few days before opening it. The smell is a trigger for me. More on that later. I also believe playing video games, watching movies, and spending too much time on the computer make our brain (our brain *muscle*) weak. Aka, brain dead.

As I had mentioned earlier I had to let learning the harp go and took up Portuguese instead. My RA and acromegaly have been taking their toll. My hands continue to swell, and my joints are painful. My fingers keep locking up (trigger finger). It does make me sad, but as I mentioned earlier, there are some things we may not be able to do. We cannot focus on that. Instead, find something else that brings you joy. So, Portuguese is pretty cool. Since I did learn Spanish about 16 years ago, and that has helped big time. Even so, it is no easy task! My memory is so compromised it takes so much repetition. Oh well, little by little.

Other Ways to Help Combat the Memory Issue

- **Write it Down**

Sounds simple enough, right? But, I even forget to write things down sometimes or, I forget where I put the list. Have a clipboard with lined paper, or a notebook that is specifically for your "to-do" list. Write everything down, and I mean everything. Everything from "order groceries online" to "wash a load of laundry today." (Oh shoot, that reminds me, I have to throw a load of towels in the washing machine. I'm serious! Hey, I never said I perfected this whole list idea. It's a work in progress.)

- **Keep a Separate List of Groceries**

Don't tell yourself you will remember because you won't. What's funny is I kept forgetting the list when going out with my husband. I started taking pictures of the list with my phone. Funny, I always seem to remember my phone though.

- **Keep a Pad and Paper by Your Bed at Night**

Often, when I am lying down, my mind races. Think of all the things you had forgotten to write down, now is your chance.

Or tell your spouse or family member things you want to remember. Often, Dan will say something that will trigger that memory muscle, and I'll write it down. Many times, he will just say, "Hey, you wanted me to remind you about…" Oh yeah, thanks!

- ## Have a Computer Schedule

This is optional of course, but I have learned to love Google Calendar. I put everything on there. All work appointments, all medical appointments, all birthdays, all social gatherings, etc. You get to color code everything, so it looks cool too. There are reminders that can be set a day in advance, an hour in advance, ten minutes in advance, etc. Try it out if you haven't. Reminders will pop up on your phone as well.

- ## Make Light of It

It can be embarrassing when you are talking with someone, and the word, name, or activity totally escapes your mind. As I mentioned earlier, I make light of it. My family jokes about me not remembering family get-togethers and significant memories as kids. We laugh our heads off as I hear one of my sisters say, "Judi won't remember this, but…" I've learned not to care so much, it's easier for me that way.

Maybe even not remembering some things could be a good thing. I read this post on Facebook that I started to implement. Instead of saying "Oh, what was that word?" I now say: "Oh, what was that word in English?" This is cool. Sounds like I know another language. This makes me laugh inside every time. Well, every time except the time my one friend asked me what the word was in Spanish! She knew I could speak Spanish. Totally busted.

Don't get discouraged when you forget things. It is going to happen, and it will happen at the most inopportune times.

Chapter 5
Triggers and Toxins

As you may have gathered by now, in my younger years, I lived a very free active lifestyle and I really didn't think too much about what I was doing, my surroundings, toxins, and all the other possible seizure triggers in our world. When my seizures began, I still did not know what triggered them. This comes as no surprise as not knowing seems to be the status quo. Honestly, it took years, notes, research, and questioning everything that my husband and I could think of. Only after that were we able to come to some conclusions that specific smells themselves were triggering my seizures. This is not something we just came up with on our own. I have worked with doctors that have mentioned environmental triggers in general, my brother has talked to me about a neurologist in Florida that has been advising his patients regarding toxic substances, and one doctor in particular, whom I worked with while volunteering to interpret Spanish in a clinic, discussed in depth with Dan and me regarding neurotoxins in our environment. As we were putting everything together, and figuring this all out, we began to make the life-altering changes necessary in our lives to help avoid another seizure.

Removing Household Items That May Be Triggers

The first thing we changed was our thought process. Knowing that certain smells were potential triggers for me, everywhere we went and with everything we did, we looked for red flags. That candle could be a trigger, that rug, that flickering fan light, that perfume or cologne, that cleaner, etc. We tried to become more aware and cautious about everything inside as well as outside of our home. I would like to share what we did to lessen the chance of having a seizure.

Let's start with the initial changes in our home. We started under the kitchen sink, in the laundry room, and in the storage room. We got rid of absolutely everything that was not natural. Things like general all-purpose cleaners, sprays, oven cleaners, stove top cleaners, floor and carpet sprays, tile cleaners, dishwasher and dishwashing liquids, bleach, products that contain ammonia, and window cleaners.

We then moved to the bathroom vanity and under the bathroom sink. Everything, even dental floss as the "Glide" brand may still contain Teflon, was gotten rid of. Hair products, soaps, toothpaste, deodorants, perfumes, makeups, pain pills, teeth whiteners, and lipsticks. Really, just about everything.

We then went to general products around the home. We got rid of scented candles, and aroma pots that were plugged into the living room and the bathrooms. We disposed of dog sprays, dog shampoos, and flea shampoos. We disposed of trash bags that were scented, laundry detergent, dryer sheets, and stain remover products.

To the kitchen cookware, we go. We disposed of every pot or pan that was made of Teflon or aluminum including cookie sheets, muffin pans, and frying pans.

Finally, we went through the kitchen cupboards. Honestly, we threw out anything and everything that had any dye in it: red dye, yellow dye, and blue dye. Things you wouldn't even think had dye in them such as bacon bits, crackers, and certain chips. We threw out unhealthy products that were full of ingredients that we never thought about before such as soy sauce because it has monosodium glutamate (MSG) in it, artificial sweeteners, and food with sugar. White sugar has got to be the worst sugar to put in your body. I'll talk about this in more detail later in Chapter 8 on diet.

We did our best to eradicate our home from any unnatural product. No, it was not easy, simply because I knew in the back of my mind, I was going to have to replace those items with healthy, nontoxic substitutes, which set off my money bell. How much was all that going to cost? We did eventually replace many of the things I mentioned, slowly. We did without if we couldn't afford certain things. Little by little, our home became a safer place to live.

So, What is a Toxin Anyway?

- **Toxin:** a harmful substance produced within living cells or organisms capable of causing disease
- **Toxicant:** a potentially poisonous substance that may be man-made or naturally occurring
- **Toxicity:** a measure of the degree to which something is toxic or poisonous.
- **Neurotoxin:** a poison that acts on the nervous system
- **Nervous system:** controls everything you do, including breathing, walking, thinking, and feeling; this system is made up of your brain, spinal cord, and all the nerves, which carry the messages to and from the body, so the brain can interpret them and take action.[18]

I am not a chemist, so forgive me ahead of time if I say toxin when it may be a toxicant. The difference between the two appears as to whether the substance is man-made. Since man has done an incredible job of making synthetic toxicants that would otherwise be toxins, I am going to call them toxins simply because I do not know if they were man-made or not. I hope that made sense.

Are there toxins and toxicants in our world? If you Google "is our world toxic," you will get about 264 million results. Google "are toxins causing disease" and you will get about 359 million

---

[18] "Word! Nervous System," Nemours Kids Health, https://kidshealth.org/en/kids/word-nervous-system.html.

results. Google "can toxins induce a seizure" and you will see about 17.4 million results.

People are having more seizures than ever before. Why? Well, as you can see from any type of Google search because we live in a toxic world. Environmental toxins invade our living environments, our homes, our food, and our everyday lives, yet so many are unaware of what they can do to the brain. These environmental toxins affect us neurologically, hence, they are neurotoxins.

So, we have pretty much stated the obvious; our world is toxic. These neurotoxins can induce seizures in some people. The quandary then? Not all toxins affect everyone in the same way, and in my opinion, therefore, many are not aware of their deadly effects.

"Earth, and all life on it, are being saturated with man-made chemicals in an event unlike anything in the planet's entire history," says Julian Cribb, author of *Surviving the 21st Century* (Springer International, 2017).

"Every moment of our lives we are exposed to thousands of these (toxic) substances. They enter our bodies with each breath, meal or drink we take, the clothes and cosmetics we wear, the things we encounter every day in our homes, workplaces, and travel."[19]

Having smell-induced seizures, I honed in on the word "breath," but it's not just what we breathe. It's what we eat, drink, and wear, which honestly includes almost every aspect of our lives and our environment.

The Well-known List of Seizure Triggers

When you start to research seizure triggers in epilepsy, you will most likely see the same info that has been out for as long as I can remember. I have had seizures for thirty years and the list pretty

---

[19] SciNews, "Scientists categorize Earth as a 'toxic planet'," Phys.org, https://phys.org/news/2017-02-scientists-categorize-earth-toxic-planet.html.

much has stayed the same over most of those years. However, I am encouraged when new insights and new triggers are recognized and added. As we create more epilepsy awareness and those of us with epilepsy share more of our stories and discover triggers, some of the unknowns and questions are being answered. Amen to this! In general, here is the "standard list" of the most common seizure triggers:

1. not enough sleep
2. stress (anxiety)
3. alcohol/drugs
4. high fever
5. not eating well (poor diet)
6. certain medications and changes in medications
7. missed medication doses
8. flickering lights
9. hormone changes in women (menstrual changes)
10. caffeine

Even More Triggers

Outside of my personal triggers and the common eight to ten that can be seen all over the internet, what others are out there? Here are some possible triggers you may not have heard about before. I do talk about some of these triggers in a little more detail later in the book, especially if they are known triggers for me.

1. Photosensitivity (flashing/flickering lights). Avoid flickering and crazy light patterns that cause headaches, visual difficulties, and possible seizures. For example, my mom's neighbor had a seizure when she was in a restaurant where the lights were above the blades pointing downward which caused flickering. Our last rental cottage had lights

below the ceiling fan blades, but they were pointing up causing flickering. For me, and maybe you, the lights need to be above the blades pointing up, or below the blades pointing down. Kind of confusing, but I think you get what I am saying. Someone else told me that flickering lights on a pair of kids' sneakers were a trigger for her. Something to be aware of.

2. Bright, contrasting patterns such as white bars against a black background

3. Flashing white light followed by darkness

4. Stimulating images that take up your complete field of vision, such as being very close to a TV screen.

5. It is said that certain colors such as red and blue could be possible triggers.

6. Strobe lights or multiple camera flashes.

7. Watching TV in a dark room, so it may help to keep some lights on. Low lights are better than no lights.

8. Too much computer time. Staring at a screen for long periods of time can be a potential trigger. Too much scrolling can be a trigger as well. I know we all love to scroll through our social media but limit the time and the speed of scrolling.

9. Certain movies. Recently, it has been said that the latest *Star Wars* movie could possibly trigger seizures in some people due to special effects.

10. Video games. I have never been a fan of video games. I think our kids should be engaged in much more meaningful tasks. In my opinion, they are becoming more and more violent and are possible seizure triggers.

11. The sunlight flickering through trees. When my husband is driving when this happens, I must cover my eyes and block them out. Be aware of flickering sunlight through window blinds or reflections on the water as well.

12. Constipation. When your body itself is toxic, your brain activity can be compromised. This can be diet related. Eat healthy fiber-rich foods. If needed, take a natural stool softener such as aloe. Don't take that synthetic crap (pun intended).

13. Before, during, and after menstruation. Your body is weak, your hormones are wacky. Take time to rest, drink plenty of fluids and give your body the nutrition it needs.

14. Excessive conversation. Too much talking can fatigue your brain. Rest, relax, and let your body heal itself.

15. Having long hair. This has been a trigger for someone I know. Be aware if this affects you, notice headaches, irritability, and stress. All of which can trigger a seizure.

16. Bare feet. Your feet are very absorbent. It may be best to use shoes so toxins can be avoided. At least wear flip-flops. In the house, cozy warm socks are my favorite.

17. TV. Just shut it off. We don't even have one in our home. Radio Frequencies can be toxic as well.

18. Stress. Oh, that lovely almost unavoidable word. Sigh. Learn to "Let go and let God." What has worrying ever done for you that is good? Nothing. God holds you in the palm of His hand. He is the Yesterday, the Today, and the Tomorrow. He knows all, sees all, and IS all. Take His gift of "a peace that passes all understanding" and bask in it.

19. Alcohol. "Alcohol is a very effective dissolving agent. It dissolves families, marriages, friendships, jobs, bank accounts, and neurons, but never problems."

20. Low blood sugar. Often diet-related and something to be aware of.

21. Poor nutrition. Read Chapter 8 well.

22. Exhaustion. We need to regulate our energy levels.

23. Lack of sleep. Chapter 7 has some great info about sleeping.

24. Anxiety. Much like stress.

25. Fatigue. Much like exhaustion.

26. Caffeine and Methylxanthines (stimulants). Get rid of all those powerful caffeine drinks. They are so harmful to our bodies. Most have dyes in them which is something we all should avoid.

27. Coffee. A stimulant.

28. Tea. Herbal tea is okay, with no caffeine.

29. Chocolate (great, lol). I do have a tiny bit of dark chocolate from time to time. I am actually starting to replace it with carob. At first, I was like, Ewwww. But, my taste buds are changing and I am starting to like it.

30. Missed medication or over-medicated. Keep your meds in a container with the times/days on it. I often forget so this helps.

31. Fever, colds, infections. Drinking a lot of water helps rid our bodies of sickness quicker. Being sick in general can cause dehydration, another possible trigger.

32. Overexcitement. Very person dependent.

33. Boredom. Keep your brain muscles moving whenever possible. Yet, not too much. I feel we need to find a happy medium, and that will differ for each of us.

34. Drug abuse

35. Extreme heat or cold. I have often been told that hot showers are triggers for several people. Maybe a slightly cooler shower may be best.

36. Infections such as encephalitis and meningitis

37. Stroke

38. Genetic syndromes

39. Reduced oxygen to the body and brain. The infamous exercise. Outside walks are so good for us!

40. Alzheimer's

41. Sudden loud noise

42. Mold

43. Medication interactions

44. Dehydration or overhydration. Sufficient water intake is vital for cellular health.

45. Sudden change in atmospheric temperature

46. Atmospheric pressure changes. For some reason, this has been a larger factor for me since my brain surgery. When storms come in, the atmospheric pressure (barometric pressure) drops. Our brains signal that we need more oxygen and the dilation of blood vessels occurs. As this happens, we may feel nauseous, lightheaded, or weak. Headaches may result, or even a seizure could be triggered.

47. Sudden shock

48. Extreme pain

49. Depression. A battle for so many, but there are ways to help fight it!

50. Magnesium, sodium, and calcium deficiencies

51. Vitamin B6 deficiency

52. Electrolyte imbalance (sodium and potassium), too much soda for example.

53. Free radicals. They can be reduced with good healthy eating habits. (More in Chapter 8)

54. Aspartame. Mentioned in Chapter 8 as well.

55. Environmental toxins. Much of what this book is about.

56. Music. Not common, but certain types of music have been studied as being a trigger.

57. Medications, specifically:

    a. Antidepressants

    b. Melatonin (supplement to help sleep)

    c. Penicillin (antibiotics)

    d. Quinolones (antibiotics)

e. Tramadol (opiate/narcotic for pain)

Reading over this list myself causes me to realize that it is almost my entire world. It appears that almost anything can trigger a seizure. Too much sleep, not enough sleep. Too much excitement, boredom. There is just this happy middle-of-the-road we each need to seek in our lives. But let's look over it again. Are there some things that you can control? And look at the things that I can control. What things on the list can you or I omit from our life that could lessen the chance of having a seizure? I personally have found several. Take a minute to go over the list again yourself. Try to cut out as many possible seizure triggers as you can. This will take time, so don't get discouraged, I'm in year thirty and still making changes in my life to help me avoid a seizure.

I came across a list[20] of the top pollutants commonly found in houses that have the greatest negative effect on health. I do mention many of these throughout this book, but you may consider taking a look at the list yourself.

---

[20] "Environmental Toxins," Taylor Medical,
https://taylormedicalgroup.net/healthtopics/environmental-toxins.

Chapter 6

Scent-based Triggers and Helpful Solutions

What about the seizures that people have had that the previous chapter did not list? With every seizure, Dan and I started to see a pattern when I was exposed to certain smells and toxins and when they would result in a seizure. When we were able to eliminate many of these toxins in our homes and in our lives, my seizure activity decreased. I'm not going to say that my seizures completely stopped because they didn't. What I do know is that the limiting of toxins in our lives has helped not just my health but our health. I never realized how many substances are considered toxic and are potentially seriously dangerous. Different items we were using daily, smells we were exposed to, and objects we never thought for a moment were hazardous, were just that, hazardous.

I would like to start with smells (toxic smells) that had a direct effect on me personally. I realize we all react differently but read on. This is NOT an exhaustive list as I cannot remember everything! Several of these smells have triggered a tonic-clonic seizure. Some have caused auras and others have resulted in numerous neurological symptoms such as migraines, dizziness, and headaches, as well as other types of seizures such as absence seizures.

You may be able to relate to some of these, knowing that they had affected you, but maybe you just didn't realize exactly what it was. Some of you may look at this list and think, "Well, none of those substances have bothered me." If that is true, I can honestly say "lucky you." But for many, they are problematic.

I'll explain the substance/toxin a little better. Not too much though; chemistry is fun, but not that fun. Then I will share what I have learned, what I have done, and what I do concerning each toxin. Sometimes I replace the substance, sometimes I avoid it, and sometimes I just do without it.

Chemicals in Personal Hygiene

Let's group hair dyes, shampoos, conditioners, gels, hair sprays, and mousse all together as I mention these toxins and chemicals.

When it comes to putting anything in your hair, on your head, or on your scalp, avoid any and all products that are not natural for the most part. As I researched this, I was awed at how much crap, I mean inorganic compounds and chemicals, that are in hair products! Substances such as ammonia, Paraphenylenediamine (PPD), peroxide, alcohol, perfumes, sulfates, resorcinol, parabens, and Polyethylene glycol (PEG), to name a few. Here is a rundown so you can get a little peek at what we are dealing with.

- **Ammonia**

Ammonia is an inorganic compound composed of a single nitrogen atom covalently bonded to three hydrogen atoms; that is an amidase inhibitor and neurotoxin. Yes, a neurotoxin, is a substance that alters the structure or function of the nervous system.

- **Paraphenylenediamine (PPD)**

PPD is a powerful chemical sensitizer widely used in permanent hair dyes. In a study in 2001, PPD has been linked to cancer as well as the possibility of compromising the immune system, setting off rheumatoid arthritis. PPDs have also been linked to non-Hodgkin's lymphoma (in the *American Journal of Epidemiology* in 2008). Here, are four common PPD alternatives that are also toxic:

- N, N-bis (2-hydroxyethyl)-p-phenylenediamine sulfate
- hydroxyethyl-p -phenylenediamine sulfate (HPPS)
- 4-amino-2-hydroxytoluene (AHT)

- 2-methoxymethyl-p-phenylenediamine (ME-PPD)

• Hydrogen peroxide

Peroxide is a colorless liquid chemical. It is a powerful oxidizing agent; when it encounters organic material, spontaneous combustion can occur. Odor does not provide a warning of hazardous concentrations. Hydrogen peroxide is not absorbed by the skin, but it can cause systemic toxicity when inhaled or ingested.

When PPD and hydrogen peroxide is combined, it is much more dangerous. Research states PPD in combination with hydrogen peroxide is very toxic and can lead to cancer.[21]

• Ethanol alcohol

Ethanol, also called alcohol, ethyl alcohol and grain alcohol is a clear, colorless liquid and the principal ingredient in alcoholic beverages like beer, wine, or brandy. **Sulfates**

Sulfates are chemical detergents and may carry some hormone-disrupting agents along with them. According to the Natural Society, many sulfates contain traces of dioxane, a known carcinogen that is also thought to disrupt kidney function.

• Parabens

Parabens are preservatives found in many skincare products. You can spot them easily on the product label because they end with the word *paraben*. Examples include methylparaben, propylparaben, isopropylparaben, isobutylparaben, butylparaben, and sodium butylparaben. "Of greatest concern is that parabens are known to disrupt hormone function, an effect that is linked to

---

[21] Agency for Toxic Substances and Disease Registry, Centers for Disease Control and Prevention, https://www.atsdr.cdc.gov.

increased risk of breast cancer and reproductive toxicity," reports the nonprofit Campaign for Safe Cosmetics (CSC).

- **Resorcinol**

Resorcinol is commonly used in hair dyes and acne medication. In higher doses, it is toxic and can disrupt the function of the central nervous system and lead to respiratory problems. It has also been shown to disrupt the endocrine system, specifically thyroid function.

- **Resorcinol and Parabens**

These chemicals (along with others such as Triclosan) are suspected to be endocrine-disrupting chemicals (EDCs). EDCs are synthetic chemicals that interfere with naturally produced hormones, the body's chemical messengers, that control how an organism develops and functions. Many manufactured chemicals mimic natural hormones and send false messages and have been linked to some cancers and reproductive abnormalities. Found in many household and industrial products, endocrine disruptors "interfere with the synthesis, secretion, transport, binding, action, or elimination of natural hormones in the body that are responsible for development, behavior, fertility, and maintenance of homeostasis (normal cell metabolism)." Medicalnewstoday.com

- **Polyethylene glycol (PEG), aka polyethylene oxide (PEO) or polyoxyethylene (POE)**

PEG is thought to interfere with the body. According to the Natural Society, the state of California has classified the chemical as a "developmental toxicant," which means that it may interfere with human development. It's also known to be contaminated by cancer-causing dioxane.

Honestly, I have barely touched the surface. I will say that the selection of natural safe dyes, shampoos, and other hair products is much more plentiful than when I first started my "toxin elimination." This is great!

Hair Products

Hair gels and products such as mousse need to be all-natural as well. Stay away from perfumes and dyes. Take the time to read the labels (have I mentioned that?) Aveda and doTERRA once again have great products as well as many other companies. Only recently, I bought a hair spray. It is all-natural of course. The brand is Suncoat and it holds fairly well. I don't use it often, but when I need a little lift, I have it on hand.

When choosing a shampoo, be intentional in searching for products that do not contain perfumes, dyes, parabens, sulfates, or any of the chemicals I mentioned at the beginning of this section. I alternate shampoos. Aveda and doTERRA have great natural hair products. As I mentioned above, there are many more options out there today. Use what works best for you.

When it comes to a salon, I get very picky. I have personally noticed that Aveda salons have the mildest smells associated with their hair products. They claim natural products, or at least ninety-six percent anyway. I alternate Aveda and doTERRA hair products, which have worked well for me. Do your own research, and of course, use products that work best for you. We are so different on so many levels. Oh, and did you know that God knows the number of hairs on your head? *"And even the very hairs of your head are all numbered. So do not be afraid; you are worth more than many sparrows"* (Luke 12:7 NIV). I love that!

Hair Dyes

I do not fully dye my hair with permanent hair dye anymore. I like to add a hint of purple using Manic Panic semi-permanent color. It offers beautiful, bold semi-permanent colors and is PPD-, ammonia-, resorcinol-, and paraben-free. The formula is also vegan, scent-, and cruelty-free. The color only lasts a few washings, but since I only wash my hair about every three to four days, it stays in for several weeks. My purple is a must. This is my way of sharing epilepsy awareness. I often get comments on my hair and every once and a while I meet that inquisitive person that will ask me why purple, and I share a little bit of my story. I guess you pick your battles here. I love the color and have not had a seizure triggered by its use, as far as I can tell. When I was coloring my hair with permanent dye, I used Herbatint. Herbatint is a vegan, biodegradable, ammonia-, and cruelty-free herbal hair color gel that contains only very low concentrations of PPD and peroxide. Its semi-permanent line is completely free of PPDs.

Hair Dryer

When using a blow dryer or curling iron, I do not set the temperature to the highest setting. Do not put the dryer right up against your wet hair either. You do not want to smell hair sizzling or burning. There is a toxin that is emitted when the hair gets too hot. Take a short break or two and let the air clear a little, it really does help. I hardly ever blow dry my hair anymore. For one, it's just healthier for our hair. Second, it saves time. Just picking my battles here.

Perfumes

Fragrances and perfumes are just plain bad. The term "fragrance" allows manufacturers to opt out of including a list of the ingredients used to create that fragrance, as the term is not regulated by the US Food and Drug Administration. So really, if "fragrance" is listed on an ingredient list, there's no telling what's in there. Natural Society even notes that there are more than 3,100 chemicals used by the fragrance industry to concoct these suspicious-sounding additions to your shampoos and conditioners. (ecowatch.com)

I personally avoid using all perfume and use natural essential oils instead. I use doTERRA pure therapeutic oils for great-smelling, non-toxic perfumes. They do not last as long as some perfumes, but it's easy to re-apply them. Be aware of others wearing perfume as well. In stores, subways, restaurants, etc. There is a sweet lady at church that must bathe in perfume before heading off to church. God love her, I just can't sit near her.

Makeup

Most makeup in general has aluminum in it. Avoid using such products and resort to natural makeup. They are out there; you just have to find them. Bare Minerals claim healthy natural ingredients in their products. I do not use them but am thinking about trying some of their products. I was using Arbonne at one point but just decided to stop using makeup altogether and go natural. The COVID-19 pandemic has made the no-makeup option easier.

Strong-smelling Lotions

You see that lady standing in the middle of the aisle at TJ Maxx reading the labels? That's me. I buy nothing with parabens, sulfates, PPD, perfume, etc., added. There are many lotions out there without perfumes in them. Once again, I use doTERRA perfume-free lotions, and I add a drop of essential oil to add a natural smell of orange, rose, elevation, or cheer, to name a few.

Nail Polish

Now I like to have a little color on my toenails. I do put color on, but I do it outside in the fresh air. Never inside! I breathe through my mouth the entire time. I also wear a mask, and this helps tremendously. I do it quickly and let it dry before going back inside. Winter can be a challenge, yet if you think about it, no one really sees your toes in the winter, so I go natural.

Toothpaste

Toothpaste needs to be natural. Avoid fluoride, it is considered a neurotoxin and a potential cancer-causing risk. I use nothing but doTERRA fluoride-free toothpaste. As a teeth whitener, I have a little dish with some sprinkled activated charcoal in it. From time to time, I will put some on my toothbrush to help remind me that I can have some pearly whites without using fluoride. A friend uses Hello products, I cannot attest to their products though.

Lice Treatment

In the unfortunate episode of contacting lice, do not use lice shampoo! I mentioned this earlier in Chapter 3, this was a direct trigger of a tonic-clonic seizure for me. Pick those little suckers out.

Deodorant

It took me a while to find a natural deodorant that actually worked! I tried so many! I now use Crystal. I used to use the hard rock itself and add water to it, but then they came out with a liquid ready-to-go roll-on. This works great! The two that work best for me are the Chamomile & Green Tea and the Pomegranate Crystal Roll-on. I recently found that Crystal unscented works great too! I tried the others like lavender, but they did not work as well for me personally. Crystal deodorant does not contain aluminum, parabens, sulfates, phthalates, artificial fragrances, or colors. Just try different ones and stick to the one that works for you. Everyone is different. As mentioned in the toothpaste section, "Hello" offers natural deodorant also, I just cannot attest to their effectiveness here either.

Perfumed Epsom Salts

Epsom salt with perfume added? Don't do it! My husband went out to pick up some Epsom salt for me to take a bath. Some studies have shown that people with epilepsy have lower levels of magnesium, so we thought an Epsom salt bath would be a good idea since I do use it from time to time for general aches and pains. It's good stuff. Dan saw that it had added lavender and bought it. The smell filled the house and right away I felt light-headed. He grabbed the bag and read "perfume" added to the ingredient list in ever so small a font. He quickly opened all the windows and doors to add fresh air to the house and got rid of that bag. Read the labels, my friends. We stick only to plain Epsom salt and simply add four to five drops of doTERRA pure lavender oil. Oh, it was so relaxing.

Hand Sanitizer

The smell of hand sanitizers has always been a trigger for me. There was a time I kept little bottles just about everywhere. In my car, in my purse, in the house. According to the Food and Drug Administration (FDA), only ethyl alcohol and isopropyl alcohol (also known as 2-propanol) are acceptable alcohols in hand sanitizer. **Methanol** and **1-propanol** are not acceptable in hand sanitizer because they can be toxic to humans. Among the list of possible effects of substantial methanol exposure, a seizure is what caught my eye. Check the labels of your sanitizers. Yet don't be fooled. Some sanitizer products are labeled as containing ethanol (ethyl alcohol), but upon testing, were contaminated with methanol.

Due to the COVID-19 pandemic, the US has seen an increase of 1,500 manufacturers of sanitizers joining the market. The FDA lists seventy-five hand sanitizers it says are tainted with methanol and some products have already been recalled. Certain name brands to avoid, many from Mexico, can be found on the FDA website.

This is even more reason to go as natural as possible. I threw all my cute little hand sanitizers in the trash and replaced them with doTERRA OnGuard Sanitizing Mist. I keep one or two in my car, in my purse, and all around the house. doTERRA On Guard Sanitizing Mist kills 99.9% of germs and bacteria.[22]

Food—What We Put in Our Bodies

Chapter 8 is the "go-to" chapter about food and eating a healthy diet, but here are some important aspects dealing with food, food preparation, and storage.

Always Avoid ALL Food Dyes

I know it's cute and fun to have a blue cupcake but don't. Cake with colorful little sprinkles? Just say no. Dyes are so toxic to your entire body, never mind what it does to your brain. Red dye has been shown to have direct links to attention deficit disorder (ADD) and attention deficit hyperactivity disorder (ADHD). Read the labels when buying food. You would not believe the plethora of food items that contain dye. Some quick examples: Doritos, bacon bits, yogurts, puddings, popsicles, gum, and a heck of a lot more! In the scheme of things, it only takes a few minutes more to check all ingredients. Oh, and I have this magnifier with a light app on my phone. It made my eyes and head hurt trying to read those tiny ingredient lists. I think they make it microsize on purpose because they don't want you to know what they added. The magnifying app is very helpful!

Artificial Sweeteners

Artificial sweeteners can be harmful. You can research studies on sucralose (Splenda), D-Tagatose (Sugaree), saccharin (Sweet'N Low), and aspartame for example. You will find studies showing possible correlations between artificial sweeteners and brain tumors and cancer, etc. It's crazy as one study can show one thing and a different study shows another. Personally, if there is that

---

[22] "dōTERRA On Guard Sanitizing Mist," dōTERRA, https://www.doterra.com/US/en/p/doterra-on-guard-sanitizing-mist.

much research being done with possible links to the negative effects artificial sweeteners can do on our bodies, I'm not going to use them.

Here is an interesting example. Saccharin (Sweet'N Low), like three hundred times sweeter than sugar, was discovered in 1879. It was used during World War I and II to compensate for the sugar shortage. In the 1970s, the FDA was going to ban saccharin because a study showed it was causing bladder cancer in rats. A public outcry kept saccharine on the shelves but with a label that read "Use of this product may be hazardous to your health. This product contains saccharin, which has been determined to cause cancer in laboratory animals." It was later discovered that male rats have a higher pH factor that predisposes them to bladder cancer, so the label was taken off. Yeah, so men can still use it? Women? And it's OK? Who knows, right? I'm not going to use it, or any other artificial sweetener for that matter.

This caught my eye as it specifically states seizures. In 2017, researchers reviewed studies[23] on the link between aspartame (also sold as Equal and NutraSweet) and aspects of neurobehavioral health, including:

- headache
- seizure
- migraines
- irritable moods
- anxiety
- depression
- insomnia

---

[23] Arbind Kumar Choudhary and Yeong Yeh Lee, "Neurophysiological symptoms and aspartame: What is the connection?" *Nutritional Neuroscience*, vol. 21, issue 5, p. 306–316, https://doi.org/10.1080/1028415X.2017.1288340.

I discuss artificial sweeteners in "the Sickening 15" in Chapter 8 on Diet as well.

Burning Food

Burning food can release a smoke toxin. If you burn something, open all doors and windows to air out the kitchen, and get away. Go outside, or better yet, take the burnt food outside. Some research has shown a link between burnt food, more specifically toast, and cancer. I just throw it out. Oh, and Dan says it is a "Santos thing" (my maiden name), I always start cooking by putting my burner on high right away. My mind is like, I gotta get this done. This, however, really isn't the safest way to cook. I try my darndest not to put my stove knob past 6 or 7 (10 being the highest). Being forgetful doesn't help either. I would crank it up, walk away and forget I was cooking things! Keeping it low is key. Besides, cooking food at lower temperatures may help preserve nutrients that otherwise may be lost when cooking quickly at high heat.

Teflon

Teflon induced tonic-clonic seizures for me (see stories in Chapter 3). Toxic fumes can be released when Teflon and other nonstick cookware are heated. We do not use it for cooking at all. We went through the kitchen and tossed all our nonstick cookware and replaced it with cast iron, stainless steel, and ceramic-coated cookware. Ceramic cookware can also be a little questionable. Read the materials list when purchasing and research the materials of your cookware online. Be sure that all your cookware is at least free of the following chemicals:

- Perfluorooctanoic Acid (PFOA)
- Lead
- Cadmium

Glass, ceramic coated, and stoneware for baking are better choices. Silicone bakeware appears to be safe if it is food-grade silicone and is not heated over 428 degrees Fahrenheit.

Stimulants

Stimulants are likely to increase the risk of a seizure. Any substance considered a stimulant should be avoided altogether. Stimulants include caffeine, which can be found in coffee, tea, chocolate, high energy drinks, some supplements medications, including some diet pills, antihistamines, decongestants, and guarana, a natural caffeine source. Stimulants may also interfere with anti-epileptic medications. Recreational drugs such as heroin, cocaine, ecstasy, alcohol, and methamphetamine are neurotoxins that can trigger seizures.

Yeah, I know, you read chocolate and freaked out. I did too. Moderation my friends, everything in moderation.

Grapefruit and Seville Oranges

Grapefruit and Seville oranges have been known to affect seizure control. They can affect the breakdown and the body's ability to absorb medication. I have read that it is best not to take medication with grapefruit juice. Carbamazepine (Tegretol) is an example of a medication that is affected by grapefruit juice. I have read that not all AEDs react in the same way either. Check with your doctor. Once again, read the labels of the items you purchase, just like with dyes, and make sure there is no grapefruit juice in your "juice mix" if your medication reacts with grapefruits and Seville oranges.

To be honest, I love grapefruit. I do have it; I just eat it sparingly and do not eat it at the same time I take my medication. I do not know if that really makes a difference or not, but I have been doing OK with it. We all react so differently, so always do what works best for you.

MSG (Monosodium Glutamate)

With MSG, we need to become big-time label readers! (not sure I mentioned this yet, lol) MSG goes by so many different names. Soy sauce, for example, has MSG in it. Certain brands of ketchup have MSG in them as well. You just never know! Read more about this in "The Sickening 15" in Chapter 8. I have replaced my soy sauce with Bragg Liquid Aminos. Trader Joe's has a coconut soy sauce replacement, but I prefer the taste of Liquid Aminos. See which one you like best.

Food Containers

It's important to mention here how we store our food. We do not use plastic. All leftovers are stored in glass containers. As many of you may know, plastic containers can leach toxic chemicals into our food.

"Studies have found that certain chemicals in plastic can leach out of the plastic and into the food and beverages we eat. Some of these chemicals have been linked to health problems such as metabolic disorders (including obesity) and reduced fertility. This leaching can occur even faster and to a greater degree when plastic is exposed to heat. This means you might be getting an even higher dose of potentially harmful chemicals simply by microwaving your leftovers in a plastic container."[24]

Notice how it said, leaching can occur faster when heated, meaning it leaches without even being heated. It also mentions in that article, that when a container states "microwave safe" that only means that the container will not melt. Leaching chemicals though? That's highly possible. We keep all food in glass, and we stay away from microwaving our food. I will admit it can be cumbersome to reheat everything on the stove every time. I mean there are so many

---

[24] "Is plastic a threat to your health? Heating plastics in the microwave may cause chemicals to leach into your foods," *Harvard Health Publishing*, December 1, 2019, https://www.health.harvard.edu/staying-healthy/is-plastic-a-threat-to-your-health.

more pots and pans to wash. However, in my opinion, it is safer and healthier to skip the microwave. This may be controversial, but I have read that steaming our vegetables is healthier as it maintains more nutrients in our food.

So here is a little more about plastics, not just when used with food: "Dr. Hauser was involved in another study that found liquids stored in plastic bottles that are subject to heat and sunlight passed chemicals into the liquids. And acidic foods, like tomatoes, can also absorb chemicals from the linings of food cans. Even types of vinyl or plastics used in homes or offices can release gases, putting measurable amounts of chemicals, such as phthalates, into the air over time. In the same way, plastic vapors can introduce chemicals to food, even if the plastic isn't touching the food, albeit in smaller amounts than would occur with direct contact. This might happen if you use a plastic splatter lid over a bowl in the microwave."[25]

I've said it before, and I'll say it again, we live in a toxic world. It is also mentioned in that article that some plastic makers have taken out bisphenol (BPA) as health concerns have gone mainstream about the chemical. With the BPA gone, they had to add a different chemical we do not know enough about to call it a health concern, yet.

Shopping

In general, be aware of your surroundings. Note odd smells, areas with possible neurotoxins, and the like. Although the COVID-19 pandemic has been so difficult in so many ways, I personally appreciate wearing a mask when I am out and about, and not being the only one has helped me not feel so self-conscious. It seriously has helped filter out so many smells that can be encountered when out shopping or entering buildings in general.

---

[25] IBID, "Is plastic a threat to your health?" https://www.health.harvard.edu/staying-healthy/is-plastic-a-threat-to-your-health.

New Clothes Can Emit Strong Smells

Some clothes contain the same phthalates as those in shoes. Think about it, clothes stores are full of new material, packed boxes, and plastic coat hangers. I have resorted to shopping only for short periods of time, less than a half hour! I prefer to do all my shopping online. Look for deals with little or no shipping expenses. Notice how some stores smell more than others. Just avoid them altogether. I took part in a neat clothing company called "Stitch Fix." They picked out shirts, skirts, pants, etc., and mailed them to me monthly. I let them air out before I try them on. Once I decided what I was going to keep, into the washing machine it went. I never wear new clothes without washing them first either. The smell and toxic content are just too strong for me.

Perfume Counter

Avoid the perfume section when shopping. Not only that but if you smell it on other shoppers, get away. Perfumes can be toxic. If the store is specific to selling perfumes, I cannot enter. Larger stores with perfume in a designated area are bad enough.

Public Bathrooms

When out and about, we all need to take a restroom break at some point in time. Public bathrooms are tricky. Take note of the smell. Was it just cleaned? Is the janitor close by? Where is the toxic-cleaning cart? You may need to wait or find another restroom. I find that even in a not recently cleaned restroom, I breathe through my mouth the entire time. Wearing a good mask has proven extremely helpful in filtering strong smells. As mentioned earlier, cleaners in general are so toxic.

The Soap Aisle

Avoid the soap aisle when shopping in department stores. This was a direct trigger of a tonic-clonic seizure for me. A very toxic atmosphere. You can make your own soaps or buy natural soaps online like doTERRA. I think I mentioned earlier the many DIY soap projects there are on the internet. There is a cute farm not far from me where they sell handmade goat milk and lavender bars of soap. That works for me.

New Car Smell

Be cautious of that new car smell. I avoid buying a new car for this reason alone. But not just your own car, be aware when traveling with family and friends that may have a new car, or have the "new car smell" spray (yes, there is such a thing). When shopping for a car, be mindful of this as well. The new car smell is loaded with chemicals, some of which can be highly toxic and could damage liver function, kidneys, and the central nervous system, and even cause cancer.

"The source of the bouquet so many buyers find appealing is in the various solvents, adhesives, plastics, rubbers, and fabrics used in car construction. Many of these contain volatile organic compounds (VOCs), some of which can be deadly in sufficient quantities. Others are just bad for you."[26]

- "There are over 200 chemical compounds found in vehicles. Since these chemicals are not regulated, consumers have no way of knowing the dangers they face," said Jeff Gearhart, research director of the Ecology Center in Michigan.

---

[26] Jim Travers, "Is new-car smell bad for your health?" *BBC Autos*, March 15, 2016, http://www.bbc.com/autos/story/20160315-is-new-car-smell-bad-for-your-health.

- "The danger is greatest when the car is new, and that new car smell is most noticeable. This is when components are still unstable and prone to what is called off-gassing — the release of chemical vapors, which leads to the odor. The heat from a vehicle left in the sun can make matters worse and speed up the chemical reaction. The danger is reduced over time, and experts say the worst is usually over within about six months."[27]

If you are car shopping, consider airing the vehicle out. Open all windows and doors for some time before test driving. When Dan and I were looking at a used car, we asked for it to be aired out. The car salesman kind of looked at us like "really?" We simply said yes, really. I smothered myself with lavender and let the wind blow my hair! When we arrived back, I was sure my hair looked like Medusa's. We bought the car.

Be Aware When Out Shopping

Cigarettes

Don't smoke. It's better for your health anyway. Also, stay away from secondhand smoke. I really shouldn't have to share a secondhand smoke statistic, but I will.

"Secondhand smoke is the combination of smoke from the burning end of a cigarette and the smoke breathed out by smokers. Secondhand smoke contains more than 7,000 chemicals, of which hundreds are toxic and about 70 can cause cancer."[28]

---

[27] Travers, "Is new-car smell bad for your health?"

[28] "Secondhand Smoke (SHS) Facts," Centers for Disease Control and Prevention, January 5, 2021, https://www.cdc.gov/tobacco/data_statistics/fact_sheets/secondhand_smoke/general_facts/index.htm.

Be aware when shopping and just out and about. If you smell it, move away and breathe through your mouth. Well, that's what I do anyway. It's amazing how quickly secondhand smoke can trigger a headache for me. Even outside! The other day, we went to a park to go biking and as we were getting Violet's bike cart ready, I started getting a headache. Dan noticed the smoke from a neighboring car. Makes me sad and frustrated at the same time. I can understand if someone smokes in their home or in their car with closed windows, but to expose others to the toxic smoke emitted from their cigarette? I still have a hard time with this.

Gas Scents

It's hard to pinpoint gas smells in general. Be aware of possible gases such as propane, and sewer gas leaks. Any odd smell in a building is a possible seizure trigger for me.

Exhaust Fumes

When walking through parking lots, be aware of running vehicles and exhaust. This was a direct cause of one of my tonic-clonic seizures (story in Chapter 3).

When using a bank's drive-up service, keep your window up and only lower it to retrieve the container/tube and put it back. This is what I must do. The cars lined up at the drive-thru usually keep their cars running and the exhaust fumes can be overwhelming. I choose the line to the outside, so I am not in the middle of two lines and maybe I can get a little extra fresh air while I am at it. I shut off my car engine since I do not want to add to the circulating exhaust. I do what I have to do as quickly as I can, and I am out of there.

New Rugs

Chemicals used in some new carpets, carpet pads and the adhesives used to install them can harm your health. Some of these chemicals and glues are made with volatile organic compounds (VOCs), which emit odors and pollutants.[29]

The most common type of carpet and area rug that most consumers purchase are synthetic, not organic like wool carpet or sea-grass carpet. Synthetic carpets and area rugs are made from nylon fibers with polypropylene backing. Of the chemicals released from carpet and area rugs, the most notable are two; styrene[30] and 4-phenylcyclohexene[31] (4-PC). These primarily come from the latex backing used on ninety-five percent of carpets. The 4-PC chemical is produced as an undesirable product during the manufacturing of styrene-butadiene rubber (SBR) latex, an adhesive used to bind carpets. The chemical is among the most frequently occurring semi-volatile organic contaminants emitted by SBR-backed carpets and area rugs and is the major VOC responsible for their "new" smell. The adhesive used to affix the carpet to the floor typically contains benzene[32] and toluene,[33] some of the more harmful VOCs.

According to this report[34] from the EPA on indoor air quality and VOC's health effects may include:

---

[29] "Carpets," American Lung Association, February 12, 2020, https://www.lung.org/clean-air/at-home/indoor-air-pollutants/carpets.

[30] "Styrene," National Institute of Environmental Health Services, March 23, 2021, https://www.niehs.nih.gov/health/topics/agents/styrene/index.cfm.

[31] M. J. Beekman, et al., "4-Phenylcyclohexene: 2-week inhalation toxicity and neurotoxicity studies in swiss-webster mice," Food and Chemical Toxicology, vol. 34, issue 9, September 1996, pages 873–881, https://doi.org/10.1016/S0278-6915(96)80368-1.

[32] Roy Harrison, et al., "Benzene," WHO Guidelines for Indoor Air Quality: Selected Pollutants (World Health Organization, Geneva, 2010), https://www.ncbi.nlm.nih.gov/books/NBK138708/.

[33] "Public Health Statements," Agency for Toxic Substances and Disease Registry, February 10, 2021, https://www.atsdr.cdc.gov/phs/phs.asp?id=159&tid=29.

[34] "4 Icky Chemicals on Your Brand New Carpet: Do This Right Away," Barefoot Organic Carpet Care, August 22, 2019, https://www.barefooto.com/blog/4-icky-chemicals-on-your-brand-new-carpet-do-this-right-away.

- Eye, nose, and throat irritation
- Headaches, loss of coordination, and nausea
- Damage to the liver, kidney, and central nervous system
- Some can cause cancer in animals, some are suspected or known to cause cancer in humans.

And contain these key signs and symptoms:

- conjunctival irritation
- nose and throat discomfort
- headache
- allergic skin reaction
- Dyspnea (labored breathing)
- declines in serum cholinesterase levels (a substance that helps our nervous system work properly)
- nausea
- Emesis (vomiting)
- Epistaxis (nose bleeds)
- fatigue
- dizziness

We need to add seizures to that list. Although I did not have a seizure from a new rug, I will say that it caused a severe headache and aura. A few years ago, we bought a new area rug. I was so excited. We rolled it up and sandwiched it between the very back of the car to the back of the driver's headrest, and off we went. I started getting a headache after just a minute and it was increasing in pain by the second. Yes, the windows were up. It was cold outside! Even so, the windows went down, and my gloves went on.

We of course aired it outside for a couple of days before laying it down.

I have a dear friend that called me about two years ago. He knew I was writing this book and was concerned because his mom had just had a seizure. His mom was about sixty years old. She had never had a seizure before. As we talked about all possible triggers, I asked tons of questions such as if there were any changes in her eating habits, higher stress levels, new health diagnosis, new medication, increased stress, new pets, new car, or a new rug. All were answered no except the new rug. She had just moved into a new home with brand-new carpeting. I told him to open all the doors and windows to allow the airing of the rugs and the home in general. I realize we cannot be 100% sure of the rug being the actual trigger. But could it have been? Could it also have been the new paint in the home? The new home construction in general? Yes, I believe so.

Carpet manufacturers recommend seventy-two hours of airing out before installation. Open windows and doors when installing as well. A natural way to help get rid of carpet odors as well is to sprinkle baking soda on the carpet, let it set overnight, and vacuum it in the morning.

Consider choosing nontoxic rugs with natural fibers such as wool, jute, sisal, and organic cotton.

On a side note, I would not walk barefoot on a new carpet for a while. The likelihood of absorbing toxic chemicals through the feet is low, but it's not zero either. In general, the rate of absorption of chemicals through the skin from fastest to slowest:

1. Scrotal
2. Forehead
3. Armpit
4. Scalp
5. Back and abdomen

6. Palm and sole of the foot

Pet products

Pet products can be toxic not only to you but to your pet as well. Avoid all pet shampoos that have perfumes and dyes. This especially includes shampoos to deter fleas. I really include dog shampoos in the same bowl of toxicity as I do our own shampoos. What is toxic to us most likely is toxic to them.

The prevalence of canine epilepsy is estimated to be between 0.5%–5.7%. This means that as many as one in twenty dogs may experience a seizure in their lifetime.[35]

The most common cause of seizures in dogs? Idiopathic epilepsy (they have no idea). Sound familiar? We have choices to make about what can affect our pets. They have no choice. All that is mentioned herein in this book (most anyway) can be directly relevant to them. So once again, read the labels of shampoo products for dogs. When I take Violet to her spa day, I ask for non-smelling, all-natural, hypoallergenic shampoo. Most have this as an option. If not, I will go somewhere else. Even with natural dog shampoos, make sure ingredients do not include:

1. Parabens
2. Sulfates
3. Phthalates
4. Dyes
5. Soaps
6. Perfumes

I have heard about Earth-bath products for pets, but I have not tried them yet so I cannot attest to the products. The

---

[35] Dr. Lisa Lipitz, "Dog Seizure Signs," Metropolitan Veterinary Associates, https://metro-vet.com/dog-seizure-signs/.

ingredients are claimed to be natural and do not have the toxic chemicals mentioned above.

Let me throw food in here too (no dyes) and go as natural as possible. I keep telling myself that one day, I will make her food myself. I need to do it and quit talking right?!

Tick and Flea Medicine for Pets

For years I have used the little plastic tube filled with tick oil and we would put it on the back of our dog's neck and run it down the spine to the tail. If you still use this method, don't kiss them, hug them, or love on them for a few days. Let the medicine be absorbed so you do not have direct contact with it. Let someone else apply it also, not you. Or, do not use this method at all, which is my suggestion.

We now use the pill form. I feel this is much safer. We need to take care of our fur babies. I tried the natural oil-based flea and tick collar and bathing our dog in apple cider vinegar and water solution. It was okay, but not my favorite choice. Try it though, and see if it works for your dog. When our dog did have fleas, we bought that flea comb and combed them out the best we could. We had to do this several times.

Flea Spray

In the unfortunate situation of fleas in the house, do not use flea spray! Well, at least not the individual dealing with seizures. This was a direct tonic-clonic seizure trigger for me (story in Chapter 3). If spraying is the only remaining option, let it be done by someone else. Open all doors and windows. You need to be out of the house and far away if possible. Let the house air out after spraying before you go back inside. I would even stay elsewhere for a night; I personally cannot take the chance. When one of our puppies came home with fleas, we sprayed the house (well, Dan sprayed as I waited in the car) and we spent the night in a hotel. There are so many ways to make natural flea sprays than there ever have been.

Until I become adventurous in my DIY skills, we will continue to use the pill forms for flea and tick prevention.

General Products

Cleaning Supplies

Let's lump all cleaning supplies into one big toxic pile. Avoid them all. Use natural ingredients like baking soda and vinegar as laundry detergent substitutes. I add a drop of doTERRA "Purify" in my laundry to get that extra clean smell. Add your choice of essential oil for different clothes and towels. I know it sounds like I'm selling doTERRA, but I'm not. I am, however, selling the benefits of the products that they offer. I use their cleaning solution for my bathroom as well as their liquid hand soap. I also use vinegar to clean windows and kitchen appliances. I am sure there are numerous DIY natural cleaning concoctions you can make. Give them a try!

Bug sprays are toxic. You should not be the one spraying for bugs. If spraying needs to be done, get out of the house. Open all doors and windows for ventilation. Keeping a naturally clean house can help avoid the need for bug spraying. I spray a mixture of doTERRA peppermint oil and water around windows and doors to keep out spiders. Yes, I have a little arachnophobia. Since we have been renting for the last year or so, we have had to concede to bug spraying in and around the property by a professional company. We called the company ahead of time to inquire about natural bug sprays. Yes, they have them. At least near all-natural. Even so, we scheduled spraying when we were out of town for a day or two.

Sunscreens

Just about a month ago, my sister and I were sitting on the white sand, listening to the waves crash in their rhythm of consistency and beauty. I started to get a headache and immediately smelled something unnatural. The people near us were spraying sunscreen and the slight breeze brought the toxic droplets right to us. I had to get out, move, go to the water, whatever it took, and breathe in the fresh salty air that existed by the water.

"About 75 percent of sunscreen products reviewed by EWG [Environmental Working Group] either didn't work adequately to protect from UV [ultraviolet] rays and/or they contained dangerous ingredients. Some of the most worrisome ingredients include oxybenzone, one of the known endocrine disruptors, and retinyl palmitate, a form of vitamin A that may harm the skin and possibly lead to skin tumors."[36]

I am very happy to say that doTERRA now has sunscreen! It is a new product and I have not tried it yet. It does not contain parabens, phthalates, oxybenzone, or synthetic fragrances. Yay!

Magazines and Newspapers

Magazines and newspapers have very strong smells. The ink and the paper when new are very toxic. When we buy a magazine, we air it out for a few days. My husband fans it outside, keeps it away from me, and airs it out again until the new smell is all but gone.

Paint

Avoid it if possible. Many paints contain volatile organic compounds (VOC) which are emitted as gases from certain solids or liquids and include a variety of chemicals. If you must paint, use Zero-VOC paints. Unlike thirty years ago, there are several to choose from now. The smell is less poignant for sure. Also, use a charcoal mask. You might look like an alien, but you could possibly avoid having a seizure.

---

[36] Leah Zerbe, "Best Sunscreens & Toxic Ones to Avoid," Dr. Axe, May 4, 2021, https://draxe.com/beauty/best-sunscreens/. This link is great as it mentions some of the "healthier" brand sunscreens as well as some of the brands to avoid.

Air Fresheners

Air fresheners put toxins in the air. Don't use them. The car air fresheners need to be thrown out as well. Put some essential oils on a cotton ball and stick it in a vent if you need a nice car smell. Seriously, that works great! And of course, diffusing essential oils is great as well.

Shower Curtains

Who would even think twice about a shower curtain? Someone who has seizures, me. The smell of a newly opened shower curtain, and liner as well, reeks of toxins. Once opened, air them outside for at least a day before hanging them up. I used to use plastic shower curtain liners for years. I now use the fabric ones. You do need to buy a good one though. I had a lower-end fabric liner that kept staining. I would wash it, but the stains never came out.

Markers

Be aware of markers such as permanent markers and coloring markers. They release toxins. There are "low odor" markers on the market, at least dry-erase. I wonder why?! Buy these if you need to use markers, I am sure there are different brands. Open windows around the area when you are using them, making the time as brief as possible. I breathe through my mouth and use them outside whenever possible. Now, I wear a mask too. COVID-19 has made me even more aware of my surroundings and smells and using a mask just helps me feel a little bit safer.

Newly Purchased Products

Most products have toxins. I really can't name every single one. But it's not just the products, it is the packaging. Take a minute to think about it. New product? New package? New box? New clothing? Toxic? It can be anything from a new roll of duct tape to a new towel you just bought for the kitchen. Let the duct tape air out first and wash the towel before using it. It takes a conscious effort to make a change to live a safer, seizure-free life.

Glues

Be cautious around glue. Working with kids, you may not think about the toxic smells. Avoid them, open windows, etc. I used to be a substitute teacher for my county. I now know that I cannot substitute for the lower grades. I love kids, but the art supplies they use daily can be toxic, and it absolutely affects me.

Cigarettes

See "Shopping" above. Don't smoke and stay away from others that are smoking. Luv ya, mean it.

Plug-in air Fresheners

Although these are made to make the air smell pretty, they actually make the air smell toxic. As the canary in the coal mine, be aware when visiting friends if they use these or candles. They are certainly seizure triggers for me. Use a diffuser with some essential oils if you would like some beautiful smells in the home.

Candles

Candles can be toxic. Burning candles could be causing health risks from paraffin wax, lead-core wicks, and synthetic fragrances.

"Most candles are made of paraffin wax (a petroleum waste product that is chemically bleached), which creates highly toxic benzene and toluene (both are known carcinogens) when burned. In fact, the petro-soot released from paraffin candles is the same as those found in diesel fuel fumes and can be as dangerous as secondhand smoke.

Candle wicks can also be a source of toxins in scented candles. In the US, candle wicks are supposed to be made of cotton or paper, but lead-core wicks can still be found, especially in products manufactured in China or Taiwan. A candle with a lead-core wick releases five times the amount of lead considered hazardous for children and exceeds EPA [Environmental Protection Agency] pollution standards for outdoor air. You don't even need to light the candle to be exposed to chemicals, simple evaporation from an uncovered candle can release pollutants into the air, and touching a candle can cause the absorption of chemicals through the skin.

"The synthetic fragrances that create candle scents usually contain phthalates. As candles burn, phthalates are released into the air where they may be inhaled or absorbed through the skin. Once they enter the bloodstream, they can aggravate allergy and asthma symptoms in some people and have been found to alter hormone levels."[37]

The only candles I have in my home, I made. Which is zero. There are so many DIY recipes and videos on making candles and soaps though. I love it, just haven't made any...yet.

Smoke (fires, incense, candles)

As mentioned above, cigarette smoke is toxic, but also smoke from fires, incense, and candles for example. Something more to be aware of.

Envelopes

Sounds crazy I know, but I cannot lick envelope flaps. Be it the white ones we use often, or the larger manilla envelopes. The taste makes me sick. The glue that you lick in the seal of an envelope is typically a substance called gum arabic, which is made of polysaccharides and glycoproteins. Basically, it's best to wet the envelope with a sponge in lieu of licking it.

---

[37] Dana Sundblad, "The Truth About Scented Candles," Hayward Score, December 3, 2018, https://www.haywardscore.com/articles/the-truth-about-scented-candles/.

Carbon Monoxide

According to cdc.gov,[38] carbon monoxide (CO) causes the most non-drug poisoning deaths in the United States. Household products, such as cleaning agents, personal care and topical products, and pesticides, are among the top ten substances responsible for poisoning exposures annually. Here are some guidelines to help prevent CO poisoning.

- Have heating systems, water heaters, and all other gas-, oil-, or coal-burning appliances serviced by a qualified technician every late summer or early fall.

- Install battery-operated CO detectors in homes, and check or replace batteries when changing the time on clocks each spring and fall. If a detector sounds, leave the home immediately and call 911.

- Seek medical attention promptly if CO poisoning is suspected and if you feel dizzy, light-headed, or nauseated.

- Do not use a generator, charcoal grill, camp stove, or other gasoline- or charcoal-burning device inside the home, basement, garage, or outside the home near a window.

- Never leave a car or truck running inside a garage attached to a house, even if the garage door is left open.

- Do not use a stove or fireplace that is not vented to the outside.

- Do not use a gas cooking oven for heat.

---

[38] "Carbon Monoxide Poisoning: Prevention Guidelines," Centers for Disease Control and Prevention, March 10, 2010, https://www.cdc.gov/co/guidelines.htm.

LED Lights

About six months ago, I decided to buy some LED tape lights. I was so excited. Hey, it's the little things. These things are cool though. You can tape them on the ceiling, walls, etc. They come with a tiny little remote so you can change colors. Within about ten minutes of opening the package, I started having a headache. Meh, I thought, I always get a headache, no biggie. The headache got worse and about forty-five minutes later, my head hurt like a migraine, and I had an aura. I laid down figuring, here comes the seizure. Thankfully Dan was there, gave me lavender, opened the windows and doors, and put my tape and packaging outside. With time, my headache started to dissipate. With closer inspection, there are two caution/warning notices on the product packaging:

1. "WARNING: This product can expose you to chemicals including Acrylonitrile, Styrene which are known to the State of California to cause cancer, and 1,3-Butadiene which is known to the State of California to cause cancer and birth defects or other reproductive harm."

2. "WARNING! This product can expose you to chemicals including Lead and Di(2-Ethylhexyl)phthalate (DEHP), which are known to the State of California to cause cancer and reproductive harm, and Diisononyl Phthalate (DINP), which are known to the State of California to cause cancer."

So, I looked them up. For more information: P65Warnings.ca.gov.

Fabric Softener and Dryer Sheets

We are currently renting a little cottage behind a larger house. It's a cute little place. Really all we need right now. The neighboring house is just steps away from our front door. The dryer vent shoots right across our little walkway to the front door. I noticed this strong smell right away. Toxic? For me? Yes.

"Many dryer sheets contain fragrance and other chemicals that can trigger asthma and disrupt hormones. In one study, researchers tested five name-brand dryer sheets. The findings showed that the dryer sheets emitted fifteen endocrine-disrupting compounds (EDCs) and chemicals associated with asthma. Evidence from studies suggests that EDCs can affect developing reproductive and nervous systems, metabolism, and cancer."[39]

There are homemade wool balls that can be used to replace dryer sheets. You can add several drops of a fresh essential oil scent to the wool balls if you would like. I actually bought some from doTERRA just a few weeks ago. I love them. I personally like to add a couple of drops of both Purify and Lavender essential oils. I love it! My laundry smells so good!

This reminds me, for soap, I tried these Laundry Soap Nuts a few years ago. I honestly forgot about them. But I will be using them again. They work great! I had bought them at Lehman's online as they were distributing them. It looks as though it is a different maker now, but they can still be bought at Lehman's, or elsewhere.

Specific Stores

Certain stores, some more than others, are triggers for me.

Since the pandemic, I wear a mask everywhere! It has been so good for me. I caught myself still breathing through my mouth only, guess I feel even safer that way. Let's go through the places that have affected me personally.

---

[39] Carol Trimmer, "Why You Should Avoid Toxic Dryer Sheets," *Pure Living Space*, June 11, 2018, https://purelivingspace.com/blogs/safe-laundry/why-you-should-avoid-toxic-dryer-sheets.

- **Shipping Stores**

Avoid printing stores such as UPS, FED-ex, copying stores, and post offices. Places that use ink. The smells can be intense. I avoid these stores and my husband does most of the shipping and mailing.

- **Shoe Stores**

Shoe stores have such a strong chemical smell in them, I cannot even go near the door in case someone comes out and I am standing close, the toxic air just blows out right on my face. All that rubber, leather, new boxes, etc.

There are 4 toxic chemicals in shoes[40] to be aware of:

- Chromium. Chromium tanning is present in 80%–85% of all globally tanned leather.[41] Chromium, a naturally occurring metal and known carcinogen, is extremely toxic to workers and still can be present even for the wearer.

- Plasticiser Phthalates. A recent study by the Consumer Council[42] tested twenty-eight pairs of shoes, in which fifteen were found to have higher than regulated traces of phthalates. Phthalates are used to soften plastics, and the chemical was found in shoes that were made of plastic. Although this substance is not easily absorbed

---

[40] Juliette Donatelli, "4 Toxic Materials You Probably Didn't (Want to) Know Went Into Your Shoes," January 31, 2014, http://ecosalon.com/4-toxic-materials-you-probably-didnt-want-to-know-went-into-your-shoes/.

[41] Andreas Prevodnik, "Report: Bad shoes stink," Swedish Society for Nature Conservation, 2009, http://www.kirstenbrodde.de/wp-content/uploads/2010/11/badshoes1.pdf.

[42] Amy Nip, "Children's plastic shoes found to contain excessive levels of harmful chemicals," *South China Morning Post*, January 14, 2014, http://www.scmp.com/news/hong-kong/article/1405279/childrens-plastic-shoes-tested-excessive-levels-harmful-chemicals.

by the body, off-gases can be inhaled and increase the risk of asthma, and even cause hormonal unbalance.

- Nonylphenol Ethoxylates (NPEs). Added to rubber and plastic products during the manufacturing process, companies like GAP, Disney, Adidas, American Apparel, and Burberry were found to have detectable levels of NPEs in their products. Although stable and unreactive, NPEs can accumulate in the body and work as hormone disruptors.

- Dimethyl Fumarate (DMF). Banned in Europe in 2009, DMF is still found in leather shoes, as well as handbags, and other leather products. Used as an anti-molding agent in leather, DMF can cause skin burns and rashes when the substance encounters body heat. A recent three-month study by the Council of Textile and Fashion Industries[43] revealed 25 percent of the shoes tested contained the toxic chemical."

I usually buy my shoes in stores that are not "shoe specific." Meaning a general store that carries everything, as well as some shoes. However, I do prefer to buy them online. When they arrive, I open the boxes up outside and air them out for several hours before I try them on. If I like them, I air them out longer before wearing them.

- **Paint Stores**

VOC paints (with volatile organic compounds) are toxic. Avoid hanging out and looking for the best color. Grab samples and get away from the paint. Use Zero-VOC paints.

---

[43] Natalie O'Brien, "Toxic chemical found in school shoes," *The Sydney Morning Herald*, May 20, 2012, http://www.smh.com.au/national/health/toxic-chemical-found-in-school-shoes-20120519-1yxik.html.

• Pool and Spa Stores

These places have tons of chemicals in them. Avoid hanging around, get what you need and get out. Limit your use to more natural water purifiers as well. When we had a hot tub, we needed to maintain the water's cleanliness. We switched from chlorine to bromine but switched again to using natural rocks and mineral sanitizer. Be sure to have an ozone generator as well.

• Salons

Be aware and careful when going to a salon. Try to schedule your appointments when there is little traffic in the salon. Make sure a neighboring client is not having a perm at the same time you are there. I have to go to an Aveda-only spa, to me, it has a less intense smell compared to other salons. They are the least toxic of any hair salon I have ever used. I ask when the slow time is and bring a mask or two (yes, I often double mask in higher toxic areas). My hairdresser is amazing and works with me to set a time that may be a little safer than other times. I always have lavender with me and apply it to my forehead, behind my ears, the back of my neck, on the inside of my wrists, and even on the inside of my mask. It started to get more and more expensive, so a friend suggested Great Clips. They do not shampoo, dye, or give perms to their clients hair. The salon does not have a strong toxic smell and I always pass on hair products after the cut. I know you get what you pay for, but thus far, I have been overall satisfied.

I like having my nails done, but to do so, I take the necessary precautions. I've only had it done professionally twice though. LOL. Once for our daughter's wedding and once for our son's wedding. The specific nail salon I went to was great because the building was long and narrow with a front door and a back door. I asked if they could prop open the back door and they did. The front door was already propped open. This allowed for cross-ventilation and helped with the strong smells. I wore a mask (yes, before COVID-19). That helped a lot also. If there had been windows. I would have asked to sit near one and open it. There are some things I must sacrifice, and this is one of them.

- **Car Maintenance and Service Stations**

Gas stations and tire shops seem to have stagnant unhealthy air. If someone else is with me, they pump the gas. If it is an emergency and I find myself alone (if Dan for some reason missed filling the tank), I breathe through my mouth, get the pump started, then get back in the vehicle with all doors and windows shut. When the tank is full, I get out, breathe through my mouth the entire time, and get back in the car as quickly as I can. Depending on the gas station, I might just put five to ten bucks in and let Dan fill the rest of the tank when he can. Normally, he does this on a regular basis, and I do not fool with pumping gas. This is such a bonus for me.

Consider tire shops. The amount of chemical emitting vapors from vertical stacks of ten- to twenty-high tires simply scares me. I do not walk into tire shops.

"Analysis of the vapors that are released from tires reveals the presence of numerous compounds that constitute the "tire smell." Some of these, mostly those emanating from the hydrocarbon oils, are potentially toxic. Some, like benzopyrene, are carcinogenic. Occupational exposure can often offer a glimpse into toxic effects of chemicals, but in the case of the tire industry, there are no significant studies, although one small study did suggest an increased risk of heart disease among workers who process tire chemicals."[44]

It has also been said that "tire gardening" is a possible concern as the chemicals can leach into the soil, into the plant, and make their way into your body when you eat the fruit of your

---

[44] Joe Schwarcz PhD, "Should there be any concern about working in an environment with continuous exposure to 'new tire smell?'," McGill University Office for Science and Society, February 22, 2018, https://www.mcgill.ca/oss/article/you-asked/should-there-be-any-concern-about-working-environment-continuous-exposure-new-tire-smell.

labors. No matter how cool it looks, no thanks. I'll pass on using tires in my garden.

- **The Vet**

Veterinary buildings contain so many toxins. I mentioned in an earlier chapter of my tonic-clonic seizure due to flea spray. Avoid going inside the building yourself if you can. If not, bring oils like lavender, wait outside until the Dr. is ready, and as soon as possible, get back outside. I breathe through my mouth the entire time and wear a mask. Or I just hang out outside as Dan brings Violet in. The pandemic has been perfect in situations such as these. I like the way we can wait in our cars and the Veterinarian Assistant comes out and talks with us. Even the doctor comes out and talks with us. This has limited our time in the building and it honestly has been a blessing for me. I do believe it has been good for them as well as they get outside intermittently and breathe fresh air themselves.

The only caveat here is that I am not with Violet. I do prefer that Dan is at least with her if I cannot be.

- **Garden Centers**

Garden centers reek of toxins. Avoid this area in stores. I buy plants that are outside in the fresh air or buy them online. Or, not at all. Plants and gardening are Dan's gift, not mine. I killed just about every plant I have ever had. Well, except one. I think we named it Hercules.

- **Restaurants**

Restaurants are borderline. Some are great, while others give cause for concern. Be aware of the bathrooms and toxic cleaners. Notice if they are cleaning and spraying tables next to you. You may need to get outside for a minute and come back in. If the opportunity of eating outside presents itself, we are taking it. I love to eat out, but it is a commodity I do not partake in as much as I would like. One time my husband and I walked into a restaurant, put our names down on the list...took our names off the list, and went somewhere else. No explanations were given, and none were needed. We knew we had to leave due to some smells, so we did.

- **Workplace and Job Sites**

A worker dies of toxic exposure in the workplace every thirty seconds. Over 400 million tons of hazardous waste are produced every year, with the majority of those coming from industrial worksites such as fabric manufacturers, pesticide production, and electroplating operations.

And because so many job sites are the source of these materials, countless employees are exposed to extremely hazardous substances every day. Below is a list of ten of the most hazardous chemicals found in the workplace and their associated health risks.[45]

1. **Arsenic.** Solid state. Found in agriculture, wood preservatives, glass production, and electronics. Health risks include cancer, respiratory and circulatory problems, and damage to the nervous system.

2. **Lead.** Solid state. Often found near mining sites as well as in car batteries, roofing materials, statues, electronics, ammunition, sailboats, and scuba diving gear. Health risks include anemia, brain damage, kidney disease, and birth defects.

3. **Benzene.** Liquid state. Found in crude oil and gas. Benzene is also used to make plastics, detergents, pesticides, and other chemicals. Benzene is produced naturally by volcanoes and forest fires.

---

[45] "10 Most Hazardous Chemicals in the Workplace," National Environmental Trainers, https://www.natlenvtrainers.com/blog/article/top-10-most-hazardous-chemicals-in-the-workplace.

Health risks include bone marrow damage, anemia, excessive bleeding, and a weakened immune system.

4. **Chromium.** Solid state. In the workplace, chromium is often mixed with other metals to make alloys and stainless steel. Chromium is also used as a coating to prevent rust on metallic surfaces. Health risks include asthma, respiratory irritation, cancer, and damage to the eyes, eardrums, kidneys, and liver.

5. **Toluene.** Liquid state. Found in paint thinners, nail polish removers, glues, correction fluids (White-Out), explosives, printing, leather tanning, inks, and stain removers. Health risks include dizziness and confusion, anxiety, muscle fatigue, insomnia, numbness, dermatitis, liver, and kidney damage.

6. **Cadmium.** Solid state. Found in rechargeable batteries, coatings, solar cells, pigments, plastic stabilizers, and plating. Health risks include Flu-like symptoms, lung and respiratory damage, kidney disease, bone disease, cancer, and damage to the neurological, reproductive, and gastrointestinal systems.

7. **Zinc.** Solid state. Found in pipe organs, auto parts, sensing devices, sunblock, ointments, concrete, and paint. Also used to form alloys with other types of metals. Health risks include nausea, vomiting, cramps, diarrhea, headaches, kidney, and stomach problems.

8. **Mercury.** Liquid state. Found in measuring instruments such as thermometers and barometers, fluorescent lamps, mercury vapor lamps, dental fillings, telescopes, cosmetics, and vaccines. Health risks include damage to the nervous system, digestive system, immune system, lungs, thyroid, kidneys, memory loss, insomnia, tremors, neuromuscular changes, and paralysis.

9. **Pesticides.** Solid, liquid, and gas states. While not a chemical, many workplaces such as agriculture and pesticide production plants contain a presence of pesticides that are used for pest control. Health risks include blindness, rashes, blisters, nausea, diarrhea, respiratory problems, cancer, asthma, seizures, and Parkinson's disease.

10. **E-Waste.** Solid, liquid, and gas states. Like pesticides, electronic waste is not a chemical but rather a collection of harmful chemicals found in and around disposed of appliances such as televisions, refrigerators, microwaves, computers, and other household appliances. Health risks include inflammation, oxidative stress, cardiovascular disease, DNA damage, kidney damage, damage to the nervous system, and cancer.

Consider not only the jobs associated with the above chemicals but the products that those chemicals make as well as the individuals having to work with those products. Now, consider you going into stores that house these products and then taking the products home. Try to do everything you can to protect yourself and your family. I know we are.

Chapter 7
Additional Helpful Ideas

In addition to the things I have mentioned already to avoid possible seizure triggers, what else can you do? Here are some ideas.

Bring a Canary

For those of you familiar with the saying "The canary in the coal mine," this makes sense. For others, let me explain it really quickly. Miners would carry a caged canary down into the mine tunnels. If dangerous gases such as carbon monoxide collect in the mine, the gases would kill the canary before killing the miners. This provided a warning for the miners to exit the tunnels immediately. For me, my husband is the canary. He is cautious of smells and other possible triggers and alerts me to go outside or get away from the area as soon as possible. Go with people that know about your triggers whenever possible, or at least let the people you are with know of possible triggers.

Use an Air Purifier

I bought an air-purifier necklace that I hang around my neck. I used this almost all the time during my medication changes and adjustments. I am very thankful I do not have to use it daily. It's not the most fashionable item in my wardrobe. However, they are cuter and smaller than they were twenty-five years ago! I do believe getting to a point of medication regulation has helped me tremendously here. I do take it with me, but just do not wear it all the time. If I am going somewhere new, I generally use it.

Lava Stones Necklace or Bracelet

Wear a Lava Stones necklace or bracelet and put essential oils on it. I recently purchased a lava stone bracelet, and it held the oil smell longer. It lasted at least two hours for me. With a regular application of essential oils on my skin, that aroma might last about fifteen to twenty minutes. I like the way I can just put the bracelet up to my nose and take a good ol' sniff. It is less noticeable than pulling out a bottle of oil and putting it up to my nose. Of course, there may be times you need a stronger dose of oil, then, by all means, pull out that bottle.

There are some essential oils that are *not* recommended if you have epilepsy as they could possibly trigger a seizure: rosemary, fennel, sage, eucalyptus, hyssop, wormwood, camphor, and spike lavender. I personally have not noticed eucalyptus as being a trigger for me. Once again, we all react differently.

Blue Sunglasses and Computer Glasses

Blue sunglasses, or lenses with a cobalt blue tint, are thought to be useful in the treatment of patients with photosensitive epilepsy. Blue sunglasses have been reported to help suppress photoparoxysmal responses (PPRs). PPR is also referred to as photosensitivity and is defined as the abnormal appearance of cortical spikes or spike and wave discharges on an electroencephalogram (EEG) in response to intermittent light stimulation (Doose and Waltz, 1993).[46] If you have photosensitive epilepsy, I strongly recommend wearing blue sunglasses. I bought a pair. Sometimes exact triggers cannot be pinpointed, so we decided I should just wear them to be safer. I do like them. They actually help with decreasing the reflection off of the white snow when I am teaching skiing.

I also wear blue light-filtering computer glasses. Although there is controversy as to their exact usefulness, there have been

---

[46]"Photoparoxysmal response 1;PPR1" Victor A. McKusick : 6/4/1986, https://www.omim.org/entry/132100

studies suggesting their helpfulness in promoting better sleep. I don't know. My eyes fatigue on the computer quickly. If they could possibly help me sleep better, I'm in.

Exercise

I know, I know, why does it have to be so difficult? But, I can honestly say that I feel better when I exercise regularly. I started a routine before I eat breakfast. Honestly, it is about twenty-five minutes. It took a while for it to become a habit (at least half a year for me), but it finally has become one. My AEDs truly affect my energy level. I am sure you may have noticed this as well. There are some days I have less than zero drive. If it is really bad, and I will not lie, I just bow out that day. I do, however, make sure I at least get a walk in that day, maybe after lunch, or in the evening. At one point, I did pay to have some classes with a Personal Trainer. I suggest this with all my heart. Yes, it will cost, but it is totally worth it. These trainers put me on a routine that was made for me! A clear individualized workout program made for me and my body. Do it. I only did it a few times so I could learn what I needed. Make sure you tell them about having seizures. This affected the routine they set up for me. I cannot do all this jumping around, hitting the floor, jumping to the ceiling stuff. I get too dizzy, and my brain feels like it's swimming in a pool of water.

After several sessions, I gradually increased time, weight amounts, set durations, and skill levels and got some great advice on how to continue to improve. Now, I continue to do my workouts on my own at home. Physical activity sends oxygen to the brain…need I say more? This is time and money well spent. If joining a gym is an option for you, do it without a second thought. But please, do not be like 80% of America. If you pay to join, then you need to go! Part of my problem at the time I was getting back into shape was that I was not allowed to drive. Getting rides and relying on people can be a struggle. This of course may be part of your dilemma as well. But don't give up, call around and make it happen. In my case, I just got used to doing it at home, and needing to rely on someone to pick me up just didn't become an issue.

Sleep Well

Our sleeping states can influence our brain activity and therefore our seizure activity. Lack of sleep is a known trigger as well as too much sleep.

Studies have shown that, overall, about 20% of seizures occur during sleep.

Most nocturnal seizures, seizures that occur during the night, occur during stage 2 non-REM (Rapid Eye Movement) sleep. It is a period of light sleep before entering a deep sleep (REM Sleep). Non-REM sleep refers to times during which brain activity slows, but is marked by brief bursts of electrical activity. Nocturnal seizures can occur at any other time during light sleep, such as when waking or stirring during the night.

By contrast, few or no seizures begin during REM (rapid eye movement) sleep, though it is not known why the state of REM sleep (occupying roughly one-quarter of sleep time) appears to be protective against seizures. This right away makes me think about how vital it may be for each of us to get a good deep sleep.

Sleep deprivation is the most common cause of these seizures. Nocturnal seizures disrupt the sleep pattern and result in increased drowsiness during the day. Like a domino effect, daytime drowsiness can then increase the likelihood of a daytime seizure.

Here are some recommendations for a night of better sleep:

- Try to sleep and wake up at regular times. If bedtime is 9 pm, do your best to go to bed every night around 9 pm. Set a consistent wake time as well.

- Napping is great if you are lucky enough to do so during the day. If you are, make it short. Long naps will decrease the likelihood of being tired come bedtime.

- Take a warm shower before bed. I prefer a bath with lavender oil. So relaxing.

- Regular exercise is a must. Exercise in the mornings instead of at night. Morning exercise increases the body's ability to sleep at night. Too much vigorous activity near bedtime may make it harder for your body to relax before bed.

- Avoid large meals, alcohol, caffeine, nicotine, and other stimulants at least six hours before bed. Yes, this means chocolate too.

- Consider trying relaxing activities before going to bed such as meditation, yoga, a warm shower, and putting a little lavender oil on the souls of your feet and pillow. There is a neat app called "Abide." It helps me relax before bed as well as during the day to get me through stressful times. It even has meditation to help you fall asleep.

- I have a friend that used a contoured pillow between her knees. She said that it actually helps her sleep better. Try it, it may work wonders for you.

- There is also a weighted blanket. The adult suggested weight is fifteen pounds. It is said that it can help people sleep better. Well, I tried it about a month ago only because I was over at a friend's house, and they had one. I'm not sure what to think about it. I slept well, but it was kind of too heavy for me. I felt a little too confined. But hey, you might really like it. I have heard positive stories of people using it, so maybe give it a try.

In addition, you can create a positive sleep environment:

- Avoid leaving lights on or using a bright night light. If you must have a night light because you get up in the middle of the night to use the restroom, get a really dim one, and do not put it in the closest outlet near you. Light inhibits the secretion of melatonin, which is a hormone that naturally promotes sleep. Consider blackout curtains as well.

- Have a comfortable bed. No explanation is needed here. You need it.

- Avoid distractions and outside noise. If the master bedroom has a window facing a road with nonstop traffic, consider moving to another bedroom. If this is not an option, there are options such as a dual-pane window. A soundproof window, which is a noise-reduction window, could help dramatically. There are noise reduction curtains as well. Any little thing you can do to help you sleep better decreases the likelihood of a seizure.

- Refrain from activities that are not sleep-related. Separate physical activity. This simply means that your partner needs to respect your sleep and not initiate sexual activity while you are sleepy or sleeping. Keep them compartmentalized.

Since we are talking about sleeping and nighttime aids, let's focus a minute on safety.

- Choose a low bed. Sleeping on the top bunk is a thing of the past for me personally. We all know how crazy a seizure can be and falling from a high bed can obviously be very dangerous.

- Wall lights and ceiling lights are safer than lamps by the bed.
- Keep an extra soft rug or mat, like those used in gyms, on the floor beside the bed. This may help in case of a fall.

Chapter 8
Eating a Healthy Diet and Epigenetics

You might say, "Really, does everything have to be attributed to what we eat?" As a person who has several illnesses, yet eats healthy, I say yes. Well, almost everything anyway. I personally know that my diet plays an incredible role in how my body is functioning. My illness can become better or worse depending on what I eat, or don't eat. So here are my thoughts about dieting.

Eat healthily. Easier said than done but do it anyway. How can I stress enough that what we eat affects our overall health? As mentioned earlier, food dyes are insanely bad. Red dye, blue dye, yellow… avoid every dye out there. I avoid processed foods. I am not 100% perfect on this, but I try pretty darn hard. I avoid packaged foods. I am a vegan, so I do not drink milk or eat cheese. I do have an egg from time to time. For about twenty-five years now, I have been a vegetarian. I have been a vegan for about fifteen years. Granted, there have been times I've eaten an egg as I have mentioned. Maybe there was an egg in a piece of cake at a party— yeah, I had some. Chances are, I paid for it later though.

Sweets are kept to a bare minimum. Plain white sugar is a killer, and in things, you would never even think about! Take chips for example. I saw these great-looking "veggie chips," made with spinach powder, tomato powder, and sugar! Nope, I put it back on the shelf. I buy nothing that has regular refined sugar in it. I do buy treats like dark chocolate, or some plant-based cookies occasionally, but they have natural sugar such as pure sugar cane or coconut sugar. Maple syrup is my favorite sweetener when baking at home making something special.

Being a meat eater is of course your choice. Consider watching the documentary "Forks over Knives." It has been a while since I watched it. I was already a vegetarian, but it sure solidified my staying one! The meat industry is infested with antibiotics, diseases, sickness, and immune-compromising substances. Think about it, and then watch the movie. Or, watch the movie and then think about it. Either way, watch the movie.

Drink lots of water. I know you have heard it so many times, me too. This too can be difficult to remember when you are out and about. Always bring a water jug and don't stop and get a Gatorade! Dye, sugar, icky stuff, you can do without it. Add a piece of fresh lemon, watermelon, or cucumber to your water. Be creative. They can help increase your immune system and boost your emotions and energy levels. If you happen to be out of fresh fruit, which I pray never happens, put a drop of doTERRA lemon oil (or other consumable essential oil) in your water. Do not put oils in a plastic water bottle, use glass. I alternate lemon, lime, and grapefruit oils in my water from time to time.

There are times I will start to get a headache for an apparently unknown reason. I will lie down on the couch and put some peppermint oil and lavender oil on my temples and forehead. This really does help my headaches go away. It never fails, however, that my husband will ask about my water intake that day. "How much water have you drunk today honey?" I lovingly answer, "Not enough." I am sure you know about the recommended eight glasses of water a day. Or drink ½ your body weight of water in ounces. We are all a little different, so this calculation is up to you. I believe our brains are just more sensitive due to our epilepsy and we need that water to help balance and calm our possibly overactive and abnormal brain activity.

What Can Be Done About It

Vegetarian, Vegan, Plant-Based, Low-carb, Paleo, Atkins, Ketogenic... I think there are enough "diets" out there for everyone. But which one is best for you? That is up to you and your body. Just as seizure triggers differ greatly for each of us, the foods we eat and the diet we choose can be just as ambiguous.

What may work for me may not work for you. So how in the world do we navigate our way through what we eat? Well, I can tell you my story for starters. I can tell you what works for me and the research I have done. It may just work for you as well.

We all know that everything we put into our bodies directly affects our health in some way. It has been widely said that people with epilepsy should go on a ketogenic diet. Let me start here. I totally disagree.

I know there has been some positive research about the ketogenic diet specifically for children with epilepsy. After doing research, I feel even stronger in my conviction that the possible negative side effects of such a diet could outweigh the benefits. This is a personal choice and I am in no way leading you to decide for or against a Ketogenic diet. It may very well work well for you. However, working with a nutritionist is very important. It may be a painstaking process dealing with all the counting of grams, etc.

With that being said, please consider reading this article[47] mentioned by Forks Over Knives.

This is another very interesting article[48]. At the bottom of the article, you will see links to studies done on patients with epilepsy who were put on this diet as well.

Once again, your body, your choice. The very best of luck to you as you decide to make personal changes through nutrition.

It was in the summer of 2019 that I participated in a twenty-one-day challenge to eat a whole food plant-based no oil (WFPBNO) diet. My church, Foster Seventh Day Adventist in Asheville, NC, made this challenge possible and available to anyone interested in joining. I think about forty people in our church

[47] Shivam Joshi, MD, "Why You Should Say No to the Keto Diet," Forks Over Knives, November 16, 2018, https://www.forksoverknives.com/why-you-should-say-no-to-the-keto-diet/.

[48] Dr. Sarah Ballantyne, PhD, "Adverse Reactions to Ketogenic Diets: Caution Advised," Dr. Sarah Ballantyne's The Paleo Mom, May 6, 2015, https://www.thepaleomom.com/adverse-reactions-to-ketogenic-diets-caution-advised/.

signed up as well as several non-members! It helped to have some of our closest friends taking the challenge with us. Both my husband and I did very well for these twenty-one days. Afterward, I realized that I wanted to keep up with this diet, but I also realized that I had a bunch of food in my cupboard that I did not want to waste. Since the challenge, I have intermittently used the items in my cabinet. Now, however, I realize I need to start back on this diet and not give up. Not just for me, the one having seizures, but for my husband and his health as well. To be honest, when you come from a vegan diet, it isn't that difficult. So let me explain a little bit about this awesome lifestyle change.

I would like to reference a certain book; "The Engine 2 Diet" by Rip Esselstyn. This book is a wonderful resource about lifestyle change and a cookbook all in one. You need to get this book. The recipes are great!

Here are a few movies/documentaries I have watched that are very informative and helpful as I decided to make changes to my eating lifestyle:

1. Forks over Knives
2. Code Blue
3. The Game Changers

They could change your life in more ways than you ever knew possible. They did mine. That old saying "you are what you eat" still applies today. Eat healthily and increase your chances of staying healthy. Nothing is perfect in this world, but you can do the best you can to outweigh the risk of disease.

Why? Why do we need to be so concerned about the food we eat? Toxins, toxins, and more toxins. Know what you are putting in your body.

When considering the toxins that are all around us and in our food, I really like the way Vani Hari in her book *The Food Babe Way* explains many of the toxins that are present in how our foods are packaged, preserved, and contained. This is not a direct quote, but the original list is from Vani's book. A friend from church added some extra information to help in its understanding. This is called "The Sickening 15."

The Sickening 15

1. Growth Hormones – listed as rBGH or rBS

- Hormone-dependent cancers – breast, ovarian, prostate, endometrial

2. Antibiotics – product labels must say organic to eliminate antibiotics

- 80% of all livestock have been given antibiotics
- Kills off healthy gut bacteria
- Antibiotics are in meat, cheese, milk, sour cream, ice cream, and even in our water

3. Pesticides – fungicides and herbicides

- Sprayed on fruits, veggies, grains, nuts, seeds
- Among the most toxic substances on earth
- Imitate estrogen and disrupts thyroid function
- Pesticides have been linked to cancer in studies
- When your body is exposed to pesticides, it can't fight carcinogens, and one of the worst is glyphosate (commonly known as Roundup)
- Glyphosate found in genetically modified organisms (GMOs) are linked to kidney disease, breast cancer, and some birth defects, compromise the immune system, and slow metabolism
- Avoid GMOs like corn, soy, canola, sugar beets, cottonseed, papaya, zucchini, and squash (buy these only if organic)

4. Refined and Enriched Flour

- Stripped of nutrients and fiber – "enriched" is dead flour with synthetic nutrients added back into the product
- Many flours are bleached with chlorine or peroxide to look white

5. Bisphenol (BPA)

- A toxic chemical found in food packaging and linings of cans
- Disrupts hormones that govern metabolism, growth, reproduction, and crucial bodily processes
- Banned in Canada and European Union
- Banned in baby bottles and infant formula packaging
- Chronic exposure is linked to obesity, prostate and breast cancer, and thyroid problems. Also associated with infertility, diabetes, early puberty, and behavioral changes in kids.
- Use only BPA-free plastic and cans, or better yet glass and stainless steel

6. High Fructose Corn Syrup (HFCS)

- Chemical derivative of corn syrup
- Associated with obesity by impacting two hormones
- Insulin and leptin

7. Artificial Sweeteners

- Some slow down metabolism
- Train people to crave sweets
- Some studies say they are safe while others say they aren't—but they are a chemical, not natural

8. Preservatives

- Nitrates
  1. used in meats to prevent bacteria growth and maintain color
  2. toxic to the brain and linked to Alzheimer's and many types of cancer
- BHA & BHT
  1. banned all over the globe but still allowed in the US
  2. Petroleum derivatives used to preserve fats & oils
  3. Studies have produced cancer in rats, mice & hamsters
- Propylparaben
  1. Disrupts endocrine system
  2. Decreases sperm count
- Propylene Glycol
  1. In animal studies caused central nervous system depression
  2. Kidney damage
- Propyl Gallate
  1. Causes stomach and/or skin irritation in sensitive people
- Dimethylpolysiloxane
  1. Type of silicone that is used for anti-foaming properties
     o Used in cosmetics & variety of other goods like silly putty
  2. Used in a lot of fast foods

9. Trans Fats

- Hydrogenation morphs vegetable oils into solid fats, which helps processed food stay solid at room temperature and lengthens shelf life
- CDC has attributed 7,000 deaths and more than 20,000 heart attacks

10. Artificial and Natural Flavors

- Added flavoring can come from cheap toxic ingredients like petroleum or can be made from anything in nature, including animal parts.
- Castoreum is the secretion from beaver's anal glands and is found in some vanilla ice cream, strawberry- and raspberry-flavored products as a "natural flavoring"
- Lanolin, an oily secretion found in sheep's wool is used to soften chewing gum.
- Natural flavors can legally contain naturally occurring glutamate by-products that act like MSG, an excitotoxin that makes food irresistible but can cause stroke, Alzheimer's, Parkinson's, obesity, migraines, fatigue, and depression.

11. Food Dyes

- Artificial food dyes are created synthetically and/or derived from petroleum, a known carcinogen, or from insect parts
- Linked to hyperactivity in children, asthma, allergies, and skin issues
- Banned in certain countries and require a warning label in Europe
- Worst offenders:
  1. Yellow #5 or tartrazine (E102)
  2. Yellow #6 (E110)

3. Both of the above may be contaminated with the human carcinogen benzidine
4. Citrus Red #2 (E121)
5. Red #3 (E127)
6. Red #40 (E129)
7. Blue #1 (E133)
8. Blue #2 (E132)
9. "Caramel Coloring"

12. Dough Conditioner

- Added to strengthen texture and extend shelf life
- L-cysteine made either from human hair or duck feathers
- Azodicarbonamide is also used to make yoga mats spongy
- DATEM (diacetyl tartaric acid ester of mono- and diglycerides), potassium bromate, monoglycerides, diglycerides
- Some dough conditioners have been linked to cancer, allergies, and asthma

13. Carrageenan

- Used as a thickener, stabilizer, and/or emulsifier
- Has been linked to gastrointestinal problems ranging from IBS to colon cancer

14. Monosodium Glutamate (MSG)

- Used in lots of processed foods as a flavor enhancer, but for those who are allergic, it can lead to rashes, itching, nausea, vomiting, headaches, asthma, heart arrhythmias, depression, and even seizures.
- A study at the University of North Carolina showed that those who used MSG in their diet were almost three times as likely to be overweight as those who used none.

- Names for MSG and some products it can be found in:
    - Glutamic acid
    - Glutamate
    - Monopotassium glutamate
    - Calcium glutamate
    - Magnesium glutamate
    - Natrium glutamate
    - Anything "hydrolyzed"
    - "Hydrolyzed protein"
    - Calcium caseinate
    - Sodium caseinate
    - Yeast extract
    - Torula yeast
    - Yeast food
    - Yeast nutrient
    - Autolyzed yeast
    - Gelatin
    - Textured protein
    - Whey protein
    - Whey protein concentrate
    - Whey protein isolate
    - Soy protein
    - Soy protein isolate
    - "Protein fortified"
    - Soy sauce
    - Soy sauce extract
    - Protease
    - Anything "enzyme modified"
    - Anything containing "enzymes"

    o Anything "fermented"

    o Vetsin

    o Ajinomoto

    o Umami

15. Heavy Metals

- Aluminum, lead, mercury, and arsenic – how they turn up in your body:

- Pesticide-sprayed food

- Farmed fish

- Food packaging material

- Your body can't eliminate or break them down, so they get stored in your fat tissue and eventually make their way into your bloodstream and invade your brain, lungs, heart, eyes, stomach, liver, and sex organs

- Particularly toxic to your brain cells and can cause memory loss, migraines, and premature brain aging.

- Remove heavy metals by using cilantro, also known as coriander or Chinese parsley, and cruciferous vegetables (such as cabbage and broccoli) that contain antioxidants, which increase the production of detoxifying enzymes in the body. Also, sulfur-rich foods such as onions and garlic help your body eliminate heavy metals.

Is this not insane? It's almost as if everything we eat has a chemical or toxin in it. Except for whole natural unprocessed foods, that is. Is a whole-food, plant-based, no-oil lifestyle for you? I believe that is up to you and your doctor. But, after reading "The Sickening 15," for me personally, the thought of eating toxins just doesn't appeal to me.

Healthier Alternatives to Mainstream Foods

I cannot stress enough the importance of staying away from these toxins. I do believe this would constitute a direct change to a WPPBNO lifestyle. If it is not for you, that is OK, but I pray you take the necessary steps to avoid the above-listed toxins. Most, if not all, of these toxins, have direct or indirect negative effects on the central nervous system. Yes, our brains.

Dan and I use healthier choices rather than alternatives. My cupboard never runs out of certain staples for cooking healthy.

Some Products You May Consider Always Having on Hand:

- Vitamix blender (the best in my opinion)

- Himalayan Pink Salt (contains minerals, not the iodized white junk)

- Liquid Aminos (used like soy sauce)

- Soy curls (use as any meat substitute; they come dry, so just soak them in water for a few minutes, use them for tacos, pulled pork, chicken, whatever! Amazing!)

- McKay's vegan chicken seasoning (used for many dishes, not just chicken)

- Nutritional yeast flakes (use like cheese in cooking, or even just sprinkle on popcorn)

- Vegan parmesan cheese (I make my own): ¾ cup raw cashews, 3 Tbs. nutritional yeast flakes, ¾ tsp. salt (Himalayan pink), and ¼ tsp. garlic powder. Blend in Vitamix blender (or it's near equal), but not too much as it will get sticky. I blend intermittently and stir occasionally. I put this on spaghetti, broccoli, cauliflower, rice, and really any dish that you might enjoy a little extra cheesy flavor.

- PectaSol-C (to decrease cancer cell adhesion factor, for Dan specifically).

The Possibilities of Change Through Epigenetics

I met this young lady recently, my physical therapist who is helping me with my back. We chatted a little about having kids. I asked if she had children. She said no, and explained that due to the genes on her side of the family, such as cancer, and the genes on her fiancé's side, they didn't think it would be wise to have children. I'm not one to question her reasoning, but it really got me thinking. Have you heard of epigenetics? Basically, it tells us that we can change our genes through lifestyle changes. Yes, change the genes that are passed down to us from our parents that may have hereditary diseases. We can change them!

Consider reading the book *Change Your Genes, Change Your Life: Creating Optimal Health with the New Science of Epigenetics* by Dr. Kenneth R. Pelletier. Wow! I loved it. I believe in creation rather than evolution, but the fact that our bodies can adapt our lifestyle and turn off certain hereditary risks? Now that is amazing.

Here is a passage from the book: "Our biology is no longer destiny. Our genes respond to everything we do, according to the revolutionary new science of epigenetics. In other words, our inherited DNA doesn't rigidly determine our health and disease prospects as the previous generation of geneticists believed. Especially in the last ten years, scientists have confirmed that most of our genes are actually fluid and dynamic. An endless supply of new studies proves that our health is an expression of how we live our lives—that what we eat and think and how we handle daily stress, plus the toxicity of our immediate environment—creates an internal biochemistry that can turn genes on or off. Managing these biochemical effects on our genome is the new key to radiant wellness and healthy longevity."[49]

If a family wants to have children, they should feel good about doing so. I totally believe that we can change our lives by what we eat, how we think, how we live each day, and what substances we allow in our homes.

I love it when medicine changes. I love it when we learn something new in science and can apply it to our lives to better our health and our quality of life. I feel that this is happening in epilepsy, be it ever so slowly. But it is happening.

I believe God's original diet that existed in the Garden of Eden could cure our bodies of ailments. Why wouldn't we want to make changes that could help us? I am not saying that a whole-food, plant-based diet will cure everyone of epilepsy, but I believe it could help our physical, mental, and emotional bodies for good. I am making continual changes to my lifestyle and diet, and I urge you to do so as well.

It's much easier to take a pill than it is to change one's diet and lifestyle. Most people choose to take a pill. Don't be a part of the majority.

I want to give a quick "outline" of the book I just mentioned about epigenetics. Even so, buy the book; there is so much more information than I will mention here.

So, there are seven biochemical pathways that govern our state of health:

1. Oxidative stress

- Excessive oxidative stress can cause gene mutation and death.

- Some foods that help:

---

[49] *Change Your Genes, Change Your Life: Creating Optimal Health with the New Science of Epigenetics* by Dr. Kenneth R. Pelletier (Origin Press, 2018), page unknown.

- o blueberries, red grapes, tomatoes, walnuts, green vegetables, lemons, carrots, red cabbage, oranges

2. Inflammation

- Excessive inflammation can cause numerous autoimmune diseases and health issues.

- Some foods that help:
  - o Green leafy veggies, bok choy, broccoli, nuts, seeds, berries, garlic, ginger, curcumin, turmeric, flaxseed
  - o Apples, onions, cherries, raspberries, black tea (also has caffeine, not an option for me), green tea, red wine (personally, alcohol is not an option for me)

- Avoid industrialized corn and soy products, red meats, and sugar.

- Every morning, I cut up fresh ginger and turmeric, and add them to some freshly squeezed lemon juice.

3. Immunity

- What we eat and how we respond to stress has a profound impact on immunity. Stress management is important; treat yourself to massages, warm baths, relaxation, and meditation.

4. Detoxification

- The heavy load of toxins we are exposed to makes detoxification an almost urgent need.

- Some foods that help: broccoli, garlic, berries

- "Taking 300 mg of magnesium citrate at dinner will help to avoid constipation and ensure that your bowel movements remain normal to remove all toxins from your body."[50]

- Drinking warm water with lemon.

- Taking an Epsom salt bath. I had mentioned this and how I add a few drops of lavender essential oil. How relaxing!

5. Lipid Metabolism

- How our body breaks down, stores, and uses dietary fats.

- Decrease bad fats: beef, butter, cheese, cookies

- Decrease: refined flours, harmful carbohydrates

- Increase: whole grains, broccoli, cauliflower, leafy veggies, sunflower seeds

- Increase: vitamin B6 and B12, whole grain products, vegetables, nuts

6. Mineral Metabolism

- Those with chronic illnesses often have disorders of mineral metabolism.

7. Methylation

- Abnormal methylation patterns are thought to be one of the root causes of excess cell proliferation leading to cancer.

The book also says broccoli and cauliflower can switch on anti-cancer genes!

Furthermore, this statement truly backs up my entire book:

"It is difficult enough to eliminate natural waste materials; but these days, our cells must deal with an unprecedented overload

---

[50] *Change Your Genes, Change Your Life: Creating Optimal Health with the New Science of Epigenetics* by Dr. Kenneth R. Pelletier (Origin Press, 2018), page unknown.

of toxins from our air, food, and water that they also need to eliminate. Consider the fact that the average American consumes literally pounds of hormones, antibiotics, food chemicals, additives, and artificial sweeteners each year, and that each one of these toxic chemicals has been shown to harm the brain. In addition, we consume about a gallon of neurotoxic pesticides and herbicides each year just by eating conventionally grown fruits and vegetables. (And that occurs even with people eating much less than eight to ten daily servings of fruit and veggies that they should be eating!) Remember, pesticides are used by farmers because they are neurotoxic to pests—they attack their nervous system. Imagine what these poisons do to *your* nervous system!"[51]

It's not just one thing that can make changes in our overall health. It's diet, lifestyle, exercise, stress management, exposure to toxins, and even our beliefs. There is no one pill that fixes all. Each pill we take has side effects, and the medical profession often deals with those side effects by prescribing another medication. Avoiding the pills of Western medicine may prove to be the best means of taking back control of your health and life.

What I like most about epigenetics and this movement toward better healthcare is the idea of personalized, individual-specific healthcare—specific treatment for specific people and their specific needs. We are each beautifully and wonderfully made. We are unique individuals, so our treatment needs to be individualized as well. We need to take an active part in our own health care. If I had done this, I could have saved myself years of pain. Dan and I both wholeheartedly feel this way. I definitely have more control of my health in my later years than during my younger earlier years when I did not take a more active part.

---

[51] *Change Your Genes, Change Your Life: Creating Optimal Health with the New Science of Epigenetics* by Dr. Kenneth R. Pelletier (Origin Press, 2018), page unknown.

Chapter 9

A Service Dog

Learning About Service Dogs

I have had the incredible opportunity to visit Canine Partners for Life (CPL) in Cochranville, Pennsylvania, nestled in a country setting on forty-five acres. This is a nonprofit organization seeking to make a difference in the lives of those dealing with several different types of disabilities. I feel fortunate and humbled to have met the lovely people involved with such an organization. Let me tell you how it all happened. As you know, I believe things happen for a reason, not just by chance.

It all started when I overheard a coworker (another ski instructor named Rick) telling someone about his new puppy litter he had just bred. When I heard this, I ran over. I love dogs and I couldn't miss one word or one picture! I had wanted a dog that could help warn me of strong smells so I could avoid certain areas that could possibly trigger a seizure.

I previously had a sweet puppy that was of a breed known to be smart and one that could become a service dog. As I started to train her, I could tell she was obviously not service dog material; she was afraid of her own shadow. A foster family offered to care for her when my husband Dan was diagnosed with throat cancer. What a blessing it was. We were unable to care for her as we started with numerous doctor visits. When things calmed down for us, it was obvious that our little puppy was very happy where she was. She had two other dogs to play with and the new owners loved her to pieces. Even though letting her go was not easy, it was the best thing for her as well as for us.

I just mentioned in passing that Dan had throat cancer. Not that it is something to say lightly; as it was another life-changing event for us. He was diagnosed with metastatic cancer of the right lymph node in his neck. This was a shock. Dan did survive amazingly, having gone through two surgeries. It was a miracle and blessing that there was no other cancer to be found, and the second surgery was a complete success. No radiation was needed. Praise God! Right now, we are maintaining follow-up doctor visits, and that is all.

After Dan's second surgery, the healing went well, and life started to get back to normal. I couldn't help it, I started thinking of a puppy again. This was the time I had overheard the puppy conversation in the ski school locker room. I did not want to jump into getting a puppy without vetting the puppy's parents, bloodline, etc. Now, I am not one to hand over a lot of money when there are so many puppies and dogs in shelters needing a good home, but there are circumstances that warrant the need for a puppy with known genetics. In the case of a service dog, this is to be expected.

Rick, my ski instructor friend, mentioned how his dogs had been trained and used as search and rescue, how the bloodline was smart, and how they had a strong sense of smell. I was so interested my hands began to shake. I summarized my desire for a service dog and asked if he was selling them. He said yes (for me anyway) and that he was donating them to a service dog training organization.

I had to know more. After seeing the pictures, I was a goner. They were only five weeks old when I asked if we could go see them. They were beyond cute. Their momma's name was Layla and she was doing such a wonderful job caring for her babies. Not really knowing how all this would turn out, I picked a sweet, little, female yellow lab. Rick assured me that he would save her for me. I was nervous, questioning whether I was doing the right thing. How did I know she would be OK? Will she have what it takes to be a service dog? Will she be smart? Will she be able to pick up strong smells? So much uncertainty made me question the whole idea. Even so, we went to visit the pups.

She Made It

Rick told me he was going to donate all but three to CPL, the service dog training center. He had promised me one, another one to the young boy who had helped Layla with giving birth, and one to a colleague of his. Layla had given birth to eleven puppies; however, one was stillborn. She had difficulties giving birth and had to have an emergency C-section. She had ten healthy puppies. This left seven that would be donated to CPL.

CPL was about six hundred miles from our home and over a nine-hour drive. For Rick, it was about six hundred fifty miles and a ten-hour drive. He planned to have the ten puppies in the back of his vehicle with Layla occupying the front seat. I began to admire his commitment to CPL. Can you just imagine ten puppies in a small vehicle for over ten hours? He'd have to stop several times for puppy breaks. His trip would probably be no less than twelve hours. Since Dan and I were already in Snowshoe, West Virginia, at a Professional Ski Instructors of America clinic, we decided to meet him in Pennsylvania.

We arrived at CPL full of anticipation and were quickly given a tour of the facility followed by the puppy testing. What a wonderful place, what wonderful people. I was intrigued by the whole idea of puppy testing, to see which ones would have the opportunity to be service dogs for those needing them. They tested the puppies one at a time using different props and watched their behavior. How they acted, how they reacted. It was all so intriguing. My deepest desire was to know if my puppy would at least be a candidate. I was overjoyed when she received a passing grade. I looked up and saw little paw prints on the ceiling. It made me think of how God provides from above all that we need here below. It just put a smile on my face.

Knowing that Rick had to head back on his twelve-hour trip now with the remaining puppies, we started to help him get things ready. Someone asked if I had a name for my pup. I didn't. How about Violet, someone else piped in. Yes! They knew I wanted a name that would be associated with epilepsy and the color purple.

Perfect! My sweet Violet has a name. I couldn't help but give her a middle name as well, Sierra. Miss Violet Sierra Bruns. You knew I had to include something about skiing in her name. Creating epilepsy awareness and skiing, are the two passionate parts of my life. Now I have a canine partner for life. Thank you, Rick and CPL.

For those of you who may not know, "Purple is the color of epilepsy awareness signified with a purple ribbon. Lavender, the color and the plant, has a calming effect, and one way to treat epilepsy is to calm the brain and the nervous system."[52] I love it.

How Service Dogs are Trained

CPL trains service dogs to assist in balance support, and aid individuals with diabetes disorders, cardiac disorders, seizure disorders, and more. There are several different programs at CPL depending on the needs of those seeking a service dog. I think the training schedule of the dogs CPL takes in is absolutely amazing and can be seen on their website. There are only a few organizations worldwide that have worked with training dogs specifically for seizure detection. Each service dog training center varies in not only the manner in which a dog may be trained but also in the way it may assist an individual.

Depending on the person, as well as the seizure, the dog may alert them and give them time to lie down in a safe area to avoid injury. This "alert" is not guaranteed and can vary anywhere from several seconds to 45 minutes or more before the onset of the seizure.[53] Deborah Dalziel, the research coordinator on seizure alert dogs for a University of Florida Veterinary Medicine study, mentions that there are no scientific studies to support exactly how

---

[52] Ali Venosa, "Epilepsy Awareness Day: 4 Things You Didn't Know About The Neurological Disorder," *Medical Daily*, March 25, 2016, https://www.medicaldaily.com/epilepsy-awareness-day-neurological-disorder-purple-day-379428.

[53] "Seizure-Alert Dogs: Just the Facts, Hold the Media Hype," Epilepsy Foundation, https://www.epilepsy.com/article/2014/3/seizure-alert-dogs-just-facts-hold-media-hype.

dogs detect an oncoming seizure. She also states that dogs cannot be trained to alert. I guess it's just something a dog senses. Maybe it's a change in our behavior, our actions. Maybe it's an odor we emit that the dog senses.

So what can a seizure-alert dog do? Dogs can be trained for seizure alert, seizure response, and seizure assist. A service dog can be trained to stay near the individual who is having or had just had the seizure, seek assistance or additional help, aid in putting a pillow under a seizing individual's head, and even grab their leg and roll the person over onto their side. Violet has not been trained to alert me of an oncoming seizure. She has been trained thus far to accompany me wherever I go and support me emotionally. Our desire is to continue with training more specifically with seizure assistance. There were a few times that I noticed her come up close to me as I was having an aura. I laid down on the floor and she pressed up against me. Sometimes she will come to sit near me, but this was different. Did she sense something? Did she activate my mind in another direction helping me avoid a seizure? I believe so. As more research is done in this area, I pray that seizure-specific service dogs will continue to help those dealing with epilepsy in new ways. For now, I am thankful for service dog training centers and all they are doing to help each of us deal with the unpredictability of our seizures.

The Emotional Impact of Receiving a Service Dog

When obtaining a service dog, please be conscious that emotional consequences come with it. Because epilepsy is an unseen disease, the general public may form an opinion of you that can be pure prejudice. Just by looking at someone with epilepsy such as you and me, they will most likely not detect a visual defect or disability. How quickly people can assume that you have no need of a service dog and opinions are formed.

There is a huge emotional aspect to receiving a service dog that we cannot take for granted. CPL does a wonderful job with its ability to assist new owners in not only being trained with how to work with their service dog but also with how to deal with the emotional challenges that having one brings. Even so, there are emotional benefits to having a service dog such as companionship. I like the way CPL states on its website that, "It's very easy to feel isolated when a condition limits your ability to complete everyday tasks, but a dog provides companionship that can ease feelings of loneliness."

Having a service dog also gives you a greater feeling of independence. I hesitate to go anywhere for fear of having a seizure in public. I continually rely on my husband to go everywhere with me. Although he says he would go anywhere and do anything for me at any time, I can't help but feel like a bit of a burden from time to time. Once again I like the way CPL states this, "You may feel you are restricted and dependent on others. A service dog reduces or eliminates that feeling and brings back a sense of freedom."

Consider other benefits such as increased self-confidence when going out in public or to a social gathering, as well as increased personal motivation. As mentioned earlier in this book, self-confidence is something that I struggle with every day. Violet relies on me for food, exercise, love, and continued training. I feel needed. That is fulfilling for me, and I pray she is fulfilled in return.

Having a service dog is not for every person out there who has seizures. As we know, seizures vary so greatly from person to person, triggers vary incredibly, and the ability to recognize these triggers is even more ambiguous. Having a service dog that can detect seizures, stay by the side of one who has just had a seizure, seek assistance when needed after a seizure, and offer comfort and independence is a wonderful option for many people who suffer from epilepsy. Having had the opportunity to experience what is involved in training a service dog, I have a new appreciation and a better understanding of it.

I pray that, if this is an option for you, you research all that is needed to progress forward in this endeavor. You may find out that you need an emotional support dog. You may find out that you do indeed need a service dog. There is a mountain of

differences between the two. Research how long the waiting list is, the rules for how the organization determines who receives a service dog, and the like. Often, a new service dog will go to someone who had a service dog that had recently passed; meaning you would have to wait again if you were going to receive a dog.

I had made the decision to keep Violet and find a trainer closer to home. CPL could not guarantee I would get her, and I totally understand that. It appeared to be the most viable option for me. All this being said, take advantage of any opportunity you may have to visit such an organization as CPL. Learn what you can. You are about to become family, something that should not be taken lightly.

Chapter 10

A New Diagnosis

It's crazy how life continues to happen whether we are ready for it or not. Nearing our originally projected completion of this book, and only six months after Dan was diagnosed with throat cancer, I was diagnosed with a new illness.

Acromegaly—a disease that results from excessive growth hormone production, specifically insulin-like growth factor-1 (IGF-1), after the growth plates in our bones have closed. Roughly forty people in every million have it. Three to four new cases per million are diagnosed annually.

Acromegaly can cause a wide range of symptoms, which tend to develop very slowly over time, making it difficult to diagnose. When a pituitary tumor has been detected and follow-up blood work shows higher-than-normal blood levels of growth hormone, these symptoms will make sense. However, when a pituitary tumor is detected and follow-up blood work comes back normal, these symptoms can be overlooked or thought to be something else. This is what happened to me. You'll find out exactly how as you continue reading. Here is a breakdown of what acromegaly can do to your body.

Early symptoms include:

- swollen hands and feet – you may notice a change in your ring or shoe size
- tiredness and difficulty sleeping, and sometimes sleep apnea

- gradual changes in your facial features, such as your brow, lower jaw, and nose getting larger, or your teeth becoming more widely spaced
- numbness and weakness in your hands, caused by a compressed nerve (carpal tunnel syndrome)

As time goes on, common symptoms include:

- abnormally large hands and feet
- large, prominent facial features (such as the nose and lips) and an enlarged tongue
- skin changes, such as thick, coarse, oily skin, skin tags, or sweating too much
- deepening of the voice because of enlarged sinuses and vocal cords
- joint pain
- tiredness and weakness
- headaches
- blurred or reduced vision
- loss of sex drive
- abnormal menstruation (in women) and erection problems (in men)

Symptoms often become more noticeable as you get older.[54]

Acromegaly is usually caused by the pituitary gland producing this excess growth hormone and is most commonly due to a tumor of the pituitary gland called a pituitary adenoma. A

---

[54] "Acromegaly," National Health Service, https://www.nhs.uk/conditions/acromegaly/.

pituitary adenoma is most often a benign tumor and can be part of the pituitary gland itself or the surrounding tissues. It can enlarge enough to push on the pituitary gland, the optic nerves, or even the brain, in which case a medical intervention may be necessary. It is said that one in ten people will develop a pituitary adenoma in their lifetime. I had no idea they were that common!

André the Giant, who was cast in the movie *The Princess Bride*, had Acromegaly. His real name was André René Roussimoff. He is most known for his time in the World Wide Wrestling Federation/World Wrestling Federation (WWWF/WWF, now World Wrestling Entertainment, or WWE). Since I was never into wrestling, I knew him only as an actor. His excess growth hormone production from childhood resulted in gigantism and later resulted in acromegaly. He died of congestive heart failure in 1993 at age forty-seven. So young. I have what he had. But how in the world did they find my hormone-secreting tumor? You're totally not going to believe this!

How I Learned I Had Acromegaly

In November 2011, I had a routine MRI follow-up for my seizures, to be sure no new changes in my brain had occurred. I have had several MRIs throughout the years without a tumor of the pituitary gland. Then, all of a sudden, there was one and it was diagnosed as a pituitary adenoma or benign tumor. I was basically advised that my tumor was relatively common and we needed to "watch" it. I did have the needed routine blood work (or so we all thought), to be sure the adenoma was not producing hormones as this could obviously become an issue. All ordered blood work came back normal. I had another MRI the following year, and it appeared as though the adenoma shrunk a little. I thought, "OK, this is good."

At the beginning of the year 2020, I had an appointment for my yearly—you know, that dreadful women's exam performed by our amazing gynecologists. Things appeared fine, and my doctor didn't appear to be worried about anything. After I got dressed, he came back in to chat about the exam. Everything looked good, he said, and we will call you with any possible discrepancies. He then sat on his little rotating black stool, leaned back slightly, and looked at me with his head cocked and his hand resting on his chin. He looked at me like he was in deep thought and paused. "Well, OK then, Ms. Judi, I'll let you know if anything comes back that I need to call you about."

That was a Friday afternoon. On Monday, I received a call from him. He said it had bothered him all weekend that my jawline looked a little suspicious. Really? My jawline? You are my gynecologist! He wanted to do a blood test. Not to worry, but just to check on a specific blood level. About a week later, I finally made it to get my blood tested. About three days later, I received a call from an endocrinologist practice mentioning a referral they received from my OBGYN. I had no idea why. At this visit, which was quickly scheduled, I was told I have acromegaly. The normal range for blood levels of IGF-1 is 50-317 ng/mL. My initial IGF-1 was 687 ng/mL back in March 2020. That's over twice the amount of the highest limit in that range! This thing had to come out!

As I thought about it, so many symptoms that I was having were pointing directly to this disease, and I had no idea. I attributed my symptoms to my other known illnesses, such as rheumatoid arthritis and a herniated disc in my lumbar spine (back). Turns out, these varying symptoms occur with acromegaly as well. I had severe pain in both my hands with intermittent swelling, weight gain (whew, it wasn't just my cheating eating habits or lack of strict exercise routines), tingling, and burning that would often keep me awake much of the night. I attributed this to RA, but also the possibility of it being carpal tunnel came up, which quite frankly, my doctors agreed with. I had pain in my left hip and leg, like a strong aching pain. I figured this was caused by a nerve being pushed upon by the herniated disc in my back.

The other symptoms were just weird. My jawline had grown, my forehead had grown, my face was bigger, my nose grew, my face overall was puffier, and my tongue had grown. That last one is freaky. Yes, it had gotten bigger and fatter, thicker. I remember lying in bed one night thinking that my tongue just felt big. I asked Dan if his tongue filled his mouth. I think he was half asleep and must have thought "what the heck kind of question is that?" I asked him if his tongue was up against the roof of his mouth. He said it was, and that was the end of that conversation. Throughout the years, because my tongue was growing, it was pushing on my teeth and causing them to separate and fall forward. Mainly the lower front teeth. I had noticed this but once again, had no idea why. I had had a tooth pulled when I was young, so I thought they were just falling because there was extra room. My husband Dan actually noticed my facial changes, mood swings, and irritability, and was constantly concerned regarding the regular aches and pains that I was dealing with and suffering from; so when I would ask him if my nose looked bigger and other questions, he just tried to comfort me and tell me that I looked beautiful. Dan believed that the effects of my toxic medications were causing my body and mood changes, and maybe in some part, they were.

Two years prior to this new diagnosis, I went to see an orthodontist, as I was considering getting some type of brace to stop my teeth from falling forward and gapping. They did a really in-depth exam that took pictures of my teeth, jaw, tongue, airway, etc. The doctor mentioned that my tongue was pushing my teeth forward and therefore causing separation. He noted that it was the body's response as my tongue was big and could possibly obstruct my airway. I remember asking him why my tongue was so big. He wasn't sure.

I wish I had been more determined to find out the answers. I wish the orthodontist would have been more professionally proactive like my gynecologist was. Even so, I left the office with a cute little folder of plan options for certain braces, the costs for each plan, and a little container of chocolate chip cookies. Everything was a go! I was not financially stable enough to purchase the braces at that time, so I just let it go, figuring I could save up some money and get it done later.

I am sharing this for one important reason. If you are ever diagnosed with a pituitary tumor, please check to make sure it is

173

not secreting the IGF-1 hormone. For some odd reason, when I had that first blood test in 2011 to check if the tumor was producing any hormones, IGF-1 was left out. Just that one hormone was not checked. What are the chances?

Be informed. I want you to be proactive in your medical care. God, love all our doctors; they are amazing! If it weren't for them, I don't know where I would be right now. There is nothing wrong with you playing a part in your own health care. Knowing little bits of information like this blood test could impact your care in a huge way.

If they had performed that test, surgery could have avoided pain, swelling, and growth my body did not need to go through. For nine years, this tumor was producing the growth hormone that adversely affected my entire body. Nine years of pain and symptoms we had no idea were due to the tumor. It was astute and proactive of my OBGYN to follow up on his gut feeling. To me, it was a miracle. I am so thankful for him! And I thank God for inspiring this great physician to go the extra mile beyond the scope of his field of study!

Once it all started to sink in, I started to feel frustrated with my doctor. Why didn't they check that one hormone? I mean, they did the required hormone blood panel tests. Was IGF-1 not checked? Why was that one hormone left out? Who didn't do their job? Negligence? Carelessness? I felt like I had a right to contact an attorney. Why shouldn't I? All that pain over a missed blood test is pure human error.

I sought some guidance from a friend. Oh, never underestimate the value of sound advice from a caring godly friend. His words were honest, from the heart, and so true that I must share them with you. He said: "There have been many people harmed and some have died due to physicians who did not give proper vigilance or who were distracted by other things in life. Most would not do this purposely. Some have made honest mistakes. No good way to change the past but it is important how we live our life forward. Press on with Jesus."

Wow. There you have it. I know it's not fair, and I do not know why God allows difficult challenges to happen to us sometimes. Challenges that bring such pain and heartache. "Press on with Jesus," he said. And that's what all of us need to do regardless of what life brings, good or bad, God holds us firmly in His hand. He is working in each of our lives whether we feel like He is or not. So, press on with Jesus, my friend. There is a better life awaiting us! Both Dan and I have peace with this rationale.

Planning and Heading to the Hospital

It's all crazy, but with all that being said, I had to have surgery to take the tumor out. My endocrinologist was adamant about going to the University of Virginia (UVA) Medical Center in Charlottesville, Virginia, and specifically, seeing Dr. John. A. James Jr., Neurosurgeon at the UVA Pituitary Clinic. He was familiar with Dr. Jane Jr.'s work and felt it was the best pituitary surgery center around. Of course, he said the decision was mine, but his concern for my well-being was apparent. Dan and I said yes to UVA Medical Center right then and there. I feel so incredibly blessed to have been able to go there.

I would have had the surgery much sooner but due to COVID-19, hospitals were not performing routine surgeries. Once UVA Medical Center started opening up its surgery center, they were accepting surgeries dependent upon medical urgency. My surgery was soon scheduled.

I'd like to share a little about my surgery, as maybe someone reading this book may have a pituitary adenoma that may need to be taken out. Let me just start by saying I praise God for His blessings. I praise Him for protection, peace, strength, and the assurance that no matter what happens, He will take care of me. And He will do the same for you.

Off to Charlottesville, VA we went. Dan and I were fortunate enough to find an Airbnb only a few blocks from the hospital. This place was perfect. Separate little home with a fully stocked kitchen, which proved essential to Dan as almost all area restaurants was still closed due to COVID-19. Finding that place in and of itself was a miracle.

Our pastor, Patrick, and his wife Maureen had generously offered to watch Violet for the week, so after dropping her off, we headed out for our six-hour trip to Charlottesville.

We planned with enough time to arrive before dark. So, we left around 1 pm, anticipating an arrival around 7 pm. The drive started unremarkably, with not much traffic, putting on our masks when we stopped to use the restroom. After several hours, I decided to open a Facebook Messenger room and invite my family to have a little chat. This by the way is very cool, and easy to use, and we just loved it. After joking around, having fun, and laughing, I ended the chat room and relaxed in the car seat watching the beautiful mountains of Virginia move across my window.

Then I thought, shouldn't we be off 81 already? As I noticed the next exit, I realized we had gone too far. Dan must have been sidetracked by my cloud of happiness while chatting with family and passed right by the exit for Charlottesville! The next hour consisted of U-turns and side street shortcuts. When we finally made it back to I-81, the sun was setting below the blue-tainted mountain silhouette.

When we finally arrived at the Airbnb, it was almost 10 pm. Because the next day was filled with appointments, we went straight to bed.

The following day, I had a CT angiogram, followed by numerous appointments with my neurosurgeon, Dr. Jane Jr., an endocrinologist, the nurse practitioner for a physical, and the anesthesiology team. They were all amazing. The morning after that, I would head to the operating room. I wasn't really scared. Honest. I had that peace that only God could give. I am blessed. I am thankful.

A Storm and a Prayer

Our pastor, Patrick, desired to be at the hospital prior to my going into surgery to have prayer with us. Knowing that my estimated arrival time would be 5:30 am, I thought he was a little crazy. Why drive six hours during the night? Just pray with us before we leave North Carolina, I thought. But he insisted. His plan was to leave the night before, pull off somewhere safe to get a little sleep in the back of his vehicle and start driving again to be there that morning at the hospital. He asked us if that would be OK. We of course said yes, as it would be a huge blessing for him to have prayer with us.

That evening before my surgery, a storm came through, causing a torrential downpour. It rumbled and rained so hard it kept me up all night. I wondered two things. One, how was Patrick doing? Could he even see driving in this crazy storm? Was he safe? And two, how could my neurosurgeon get any sleep during this torrential downpour? Will he be rested? Will he be ready? I said a quick prayer and fell back asleep for a few minutes before my alarm went off.

As Dan and I got into the car and headed to the hospital, I received a text from Patrick. "I'm here." Wow. Yes, I was glad to see his text and thankful that he arrived safely. As Dan pulled the car into the half circle in front of the medical center at 5:15 am, I saw Pastor Patrick. There he was, sitting on a bench, legs crossed, reading a book. I swear to you, he looked rested and as though he had not a care in the world. Although he may have appeared this way, he had to have so much on his mind.

As we got out of the car, we each put on our face masks. Such a difficult world we live in not being able to hug the people that we care about. The three of us formed a little circle keeping in mind the need for social distancing. Patrick called his wife Maureen who wanted to be a part of the prayer we were about to have. A powerful prayer to the Great Physician and an "Amen."

As we separated, Dan and I had a moment to hold each other tight, telling each other how much we loved each other. The hardest part for me was that, due to the coronavirus, Dan couldn't accompany me. He couldn't stay with me, be with me, and hold my hand. I had to walk into the hospital alone.

Along the front of the hospital was a small corridor of glass paralleling the outside sidewalk. Once I entered, I glanced back, and Dan was standing outside watching me. As I headed down the hallway, he headed down the sidewalk. Each step was almost in unison as we continued glancing at each other, looking where we were going, and glancing back at each other as we walked to the end. There it was before me, the entrance to surgery check-in. We stared at each other and gave a final wave and I walked through the doors.

I wanted him to be with me longer, to stay with me until they wheeled me to the operating room. He's my rock and I just prayed I somehow would make it through without him. Oh, how I wished he could have been with me. "Lord, be with me and be with Dan," I whisper softly.

Surgery in the Time of COVID

While I'm in pre-op, I get my intravenous (IV) line inserted, I chat with the Ear, Nose, and Throat (ENT) team, check-ins with the anesthesiology team are done, and discussions with the nurses are done, also. The final person to come and see me before we head into the surgery room was my neurosurgeon, Dr. Jane Jr.

Let me remind you about the night before. I was up most of the night with the raging thunderstorm. It was noisy. I couldn't sleep. I was concerned Dr. Jane, Jr. would be tired from lack of sleep. Now there he was, standing by my gurney. The first words out of this amazing man's mouth were, "Wow, I slept great last night." He continued, "I feel rested, I am awake, and it's going to be a great day."

As I lay there looking at him, I was speechless. I shook off my disbelief. "That's crazy," I said. "I prayed that you would have a good night's rest."

"Well, I did," he continued. "The rain lulled me to sleep, and my flowers got what they needed."

I honestly could not believe what I was hearing. Maybe as you're reading this you can't believe it either. It really happened. Think about how words can affect the mind, the body, and the soul. I was immediately calmed. I was relaxed. I was going to do OK.

He then tapped me on my shoulder and said, "You're going to do great."

As he turned to leave, I replied, "You're going to do great," although I am not sure he heard me. What an incredible man. That's all I have to say. What an incredible man.

I thought they would knock me out before wheeling me down the hall to the operating room. Instead, I get wheeled into the surgery room. Bright lights and bright silver shining everywhere, tables covered with the needed sanitized surgical instruments, nurses preparing the room for the surgeons soon to enter. Operating vernacular swings back and forth as to the current supplies, needs, etc. I am asked to move over to the table. As I slide off the gurney and onto the operating table, I'm thinking, "This table will only fit one butt cheek." I manage to lay in the center as they begin to strap me down with Velcro around my arms, chest, and legs. That was a little unsettling, but God gave me peace.

The man at my head is the anesthesiologist who puts the oxygen mask on my face. Another comes along my side and tells me I will soon be fast asleep as he administers medication through my IV. I take one last look at the anesthesiologist, who looks right into my eyes and says, "We will take good care of you." Really, can it get any better than that?

What amazes me is that the next thing I see are the nurses in recovery and my amazing neurosurgeon, Dr. Jane Jr. I believe they said the surgery was about an hour. But for me? A second. You know, this is how it will be when Christ returns. If we have died before He returns, it is like a sleep, the blinking of an eye, and we will awake to see His face, His glorious return! Hallelujah!

Due to COVID-19, Dan was allowed to spend only four hours with me at some point during my hospital stay and that was it. We decided it would be the initial four hours once I arrived at my room after the surgery. As I opened my eyes intermittently, I saw Dan. He stayed with me as long as he could (just a little over the allowed 4 hours), and we said goodbye.

I can't remember if it was the night of my surgery or the following night, but I woke up one morning with a large bite on the side of my tongue. Yes, I had a seizure. Well, I believe I did anyway. The good part is that it wasn't that bad. As you know there are multiple signs of having a bad seizure, like bruises on your legs, arms, face, and busted blood vessels in your eyes for example. I had none of these outcomes. Just very dizzy for a while, and I can only assume that I slept most of it off. About a week prior to my surgery, my neurologist had increased my medication. I am thankful for this as I'm sure my seizure could have been more severe.

Three days later, I was released from the hospital. Can you believe that? Three days after brain surgery and you get to go home. It's amazing. I am so thankful for medicine and how we have advanced over the years. I'm thankful for our doctors and our hospitals. All those involved with my recovery were amazing and I am so blessed. They are all heroes, even more so during this COVID-19 pandemic.

As I was being wheeled out of my room and down the hall, I started singing. I cannot remember the song, but the lady transporting me joined right in. Dan was there outside waiting for me. Joy. Pure joy.

Two weeks post-surgery, I was sitting at my desk a little tired and a little nauseous but desperately wanting to finish this book to get it into the hands of those that it may help. Recovery can be slow, but at least we were moving in the right direction.

My IGF-1 level blood test was taken Sept. 2021, about 1 year and 3 months post-surgery. It was 116ng/mL. Ridiculously low and completely awesome!

Could Seizures Actually Cease?

One of the interesting questions that arose post-surgery is the possibility of my seizures actually ceasing. Is that possible? Has there been any prior study of pituitary surgeries that result in the ending of epilepsy? Come to find out, there has been no researched conclusion of pituitary adenomas (noncancerous tumors) relating to seizures. Let me clarify that a little.

If a pituitary adenoma is large enough, it can cause pressure on the brain, leading to seizures or blockage of the normal flow of cerebrospinal fluid. This can result in brain compromise and possible seizures. In and of itself, however, there is no direct link between pituitary adenomas causing seizures. Most pituitary adenomas are benign incidental findings, and most are watched and followed up on with MRIs. If the tumor is large enough and/or secreting hormones, the need for intervention arises.

Yet even though there is no direct correlation between seizures and a normal-sized pituitary tumor that is not hormone-secreting or pushing on the brain, I believe there are some indirect effects or indirect triggers for having a seizure. Think about it: your body is changing, hormones are wacky, anxiety is high, hot flashes, your overall stress level is higher because you have a tumor, and the possible need to have brain surgery to take it out, and so on.

In my case, the IGF-1 hormone my tumor was producing was a growth hormone that caused a plethora of symptoms. I mentioned these earlier. I was having pain in different areas of my body in a seemingly constant state. Maybe not all at the same time, but the pain and consequences were all over the chart. I can guarantee you this took a toll on my body and mind. Stress, loss of sleep, anxiety, and the like are all possible seizure triggers. That said, let me be brave enough to say that yes, having a hormone-producing pituitary adenoma could result in triggering a seizure. Be it direct or indirect, it really doesn't matter.

Tumor Effects

I want to share what effect acromegaly has had on my appearance. I thought I was noticing changes in my face and had no idea why.

My hair has fallen out quite a bit, but just to see the facial changes, I am sharing the pictures. The hair falling out for me was attributed to Lamictal, or so we believe. I was having major stomach issues as well, in pain, and doubled over at times. Most of my pain was during the night, but it got to where I could not sleep. My family physician is absolutely amazing, and he did all he could to find out the source. Upper and lower gastrointestinal studies, blood work, and CT scan all came back normal. I decided to stop my Lamictal and go back to Vimpat. Although Vimpat makes my head hurt with pressure and dizziness, my abdominal pain has decreased, and my hair has started to grow back slowly since I made the medication change. The real culprit? Still not sure. Isn't epilepsy crazy? So many things we may never know.

Here is some new research I found. Prior research on hair loss after acromegaly treatment was rarely studied. Japanese researchers did a study in Japan on more than five hundred patients that had transsphenoidal (through the nose) acromegaly surgery, and they found that fifty-four percent experienced some level of hair loss between three to six months after surgery.[55]

What? I had never heard this. Could my hair loss be attributed to the surgery? The Lamictal? Maybe both? One year post-surgery, along with stopping the Lamictal, my hair is slowly growing back. I guess we may never know the culprit. Maybe a combination of both the Lamictal and the surgery. I'm too thankful to try and figure it all out now.

Remember my orthodontist appointment back in 2018? Well, I was ready to go back recently. My tongue had decreased in size and having some type of brace on my lower teeth to decrease

---

[55] Nicole Joseph, "Hair Loss Commonly Experienced in Patients Following Acromegaly Surgery," EndocrineWeb/Remedy Health Media, January 21, 2016, https://www.endocrineweb.com/professional/other-endocrine-disorders/hair-loss-commonly-experienced-patients-following-acromegaly-.

the spacing would be totally doable now. I made the initial appointment. I wanted to share my desire with the orthodontist and his assistant about creating awareness about acromegaly. It is such a rare illness, I felt the desire to help spread its awareness. I mentioned how his particular line of work could possibly help individuals that were noticing their teeth were separating and had no idea why. Is it possible there are others out there suffering from acromegaly and do not even know it like I was? Yes! There are others like me, I believe there are.

But once I expressed my desire to advocate for others that may have acromegaly, he changed. I realize people can misread people all the time. I'm no expert. But I felt it. He did a quick look at my teeth, and said, "There is nothing we can do."

Really? My tongue is smaller, the swelling has gone down, and there is nothing you can do. When my tongue was bigger in 2018, you offered your services. What is the real reason you have no desire to put braces on my teeth now? Because I shared with you my desire to create awareness? Did he feel threatened because I was trying to explain that this was possibly overlooked with me? Honestly, I was hurt. But, I was doing amazing at the same time. I just wanted him to know what happened in case he met a new client that had teeth separating and a larger-than-normal tongue size. Maybe he could help someone early on that had acromegaly and did not know it, like me.

With all that said, I know that all things happen for a reason. I need to focus on the positive and trust in God. I'm actually thankful that this orthodontist will not be putting braces on my teeth. I think you know why. I'm getting a second opinion.

Chapter 11

Living

Make Peace With Yourself and With God

I think the takeaway here is making peace. Make peace with yourself, with family, with friends, and most importantly, make peace with God. I read a statement in "The Acts of the Apostles" by Ellen G. White which reads, "God could have proclaimed His truth through sinless angels, but this is not His plan. He chooses human beings, men compassed with infirmity as instruments in the working out of His designs. The priceless treasure is placed in earthen vessels." That means me, that means you, and anyone else that chooses to be a light for God. He chooses those with afflictions...how crazy is that?!

We know that Paul, one of the most influential New Testament writers, had some type of physical ailment. The actual ailment is debated by scholars, but some of the opinions are that he had epilepsy, rheumatoid arthritis, or visual impairment. Whatever it is that he had, he was still used by God. How comforting and reassuring this is. 2 Corinthians 12:9 says, "*But he said to me, 'my grace is sufficient for you, for my power is made perfect in weakness.' Therefore, I will boast all the more gladly about my weaknesses, so that Christ's power may rest on me.*"

God will never give us more than we can handle. Romans 8:28 is my husband's favorite verse. It says, "*And we know that in all things God works for the good of those who love Him, who have been called according to His purpose.*"

And my favorite verse is Jeremiah 29:11, "*For I know the plans I have for you,*" declares the Lord, "*plans to prosper you and not to harm you, plans to give you hope and a future.*"

At times life can be difficult to live. There are days when you just want to give up. Days when you feel completely overwhelmed. My prayer is that when these days hit, you get down on your knees and pray for strength. At these times, I don't even want to pray, and I don't even know what to say anyway. When this happens, I say "Jesus, will you please pray for me? You are the intercessor for me. You already know what I need before I even ask. I just don't know what to do. Please tell God to help me. I just need help." When I find my life in this valley, I'm so overcome by anxiety, stress, and depression that I take a nap. I'm not going to say that when I wake up, I am 100% better, full of joy and happiness that makes me want to jump ten feet in the air. But I will say that I feel more relaxed. I feel there is a higher power watching over me, caring for me, and loving me.

There is a higher power watching over you, caring for you, and loving you.

Moving On

May 28, 2021, one year after my surgery—I cannot believe that amount of time has passed. I am grateful, thankful, and blessed. I thank God He has carried me through all of this. I am not back to one hundred percent yet, and that's OK. Even if I never get back to one hundred percent, that's OK. Recovery takes time. I still deal with pressure, headaches, dizziness, etc. Many of these symptoms may be medication-related, but could some be a lingering effect from the surgery? Maybe. We just need to be kind to ourselves and let the recovery take as long as it needs. Every day it's a choice. I am trying to challenge my limits instead of limiting my challenges!

Here is where the choice is ours. How do we live our lives? We can't choose what happens to us in our lifetime, but we can choose how we react.

I love this quote:

"There are only two ways to live your life. One is as though nothing is a miracle. The other is as though everything is a miracle." —Albert Einstein

You are a miracle. I am a miracle. Life is a miracle. To my fellow epilepsy warriors, my purple fighting friends, and my fellow survivors, God bless each and every one of you! The trials on this earth make us stronger. Each one of you is a strong tower! Keep up the good fight! You are not alone!

There are days I get so overwhelmed and frustrated. I have not hidden that from you at all. But I will say this, the days that I start with Christ, are the winning days of my life.

Live your life like everything is a miracle.

Glossary

Absence seizure: A type of seizure that causes a brief sudden lapse in attention, a staring into space, or sudden lapses of consciousness between 10 and 30 seconds.

Acromegaly: A rare condition where the body produces too much growth hormone causing body tissues and bones to grow more quickly.

Adenoma: A noncancerous tumor

Aura: The first part of a focal aware seizure before consciousness is impaired. Also referred to as the warning sign before a tonic-clonic seizure.

Autoimmune disease: A disease in which the body's immune system attacks health.

Autoimmune epilepsy: Epilepsy caused by a change in immune function.

Breakthrough seizure: A seizure that suddenly occurs when an epilepsy patient has experienced a sustained period of freedom from seizures (12 months) while on treatment.

Epigenetics: The study of how your behaviors and your environment can cause changes that affect the way your genes work.

Epilepsy: A neurological disorder marked by sudden recurrent episodes of sensory disturbance, loss of consciousness, or convulsions, associated with abnormal electrical activity in the brain.

Flare-up: Intense pain and stiffness in the joints. (Rheumatoid arthritis flare-up)

Focal Seizure: Also called partial seizures occur when only a portion of the brain is involved.

Grand mal seizure: See *tonic-clonic seizure.*

Ischemic stroke: When oxygen-rich blood flow to the brain becomes blocked.

Migraine: A headache that can cause severe throbbing pain or a pulsing sensation (usually on one side of the head.)

Nervous System: The nervous system controls everything you do, including breathing, walking, thinking, and feeling. It comprises the brain, spinal cord, and all the nerves in the body. The nerves carry messages to and from the body, so the brain can interpret them and take action.

Neurological challenge: Disorders that affect the brain as well as the nerves found throughout the human body and the spinal cord.

Neurotoxin: A poison that acts on the nervous system.

Petit mal seizure: See *absence seizure.*

Reflex epilepsy: A group of epilepsy syndromes in which a certain trigger or stimulus brings on seizures.

Rheumatoid arthritis: A chronic inflammatory disorder affecting many joints including those in the hands and feet.

Tonic-clonic seizure: A seizure in which a person loses consciousness, muscles stiffen, and jerking movements are seen. The whole brain is involved, unlike a partial seizure. (The old term is grand mal which is no longer used).

Seizure: A burst of uncontrolled electrical activity/disturbance in the brain.

Toxicant: A potentially poisonous substance that may be man-made or naturally occurring.

Toxicity: A measure of the degree to which something is toxic or poisonous.

Toxin: A harmful substance produced within living cells or organisms capable of causing disease.

Trigger: A factor that can cause a seizure in a person who either has epilepsy or not. Sometimes it may not be the actual cause (such as a brain tumor for example), but it can initiate a seizure.

Photo Gallery

Pics of Violet as a Puppy

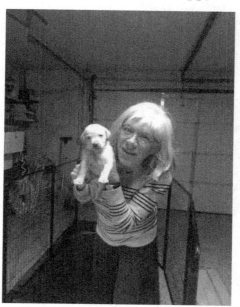

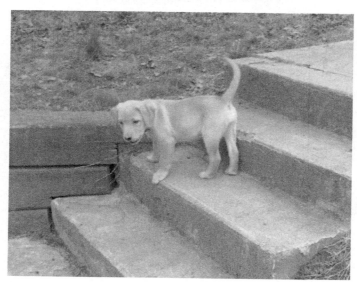

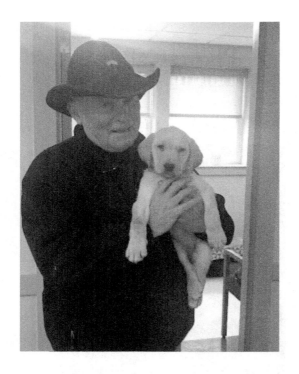

This is Rick holding Violet as a puppy at CPL

More Photos of Violet

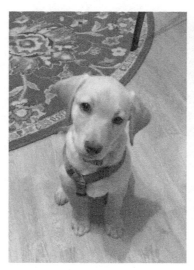
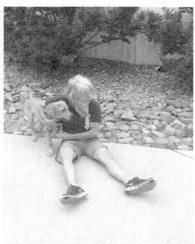

My sweet girl Violet now

She does just about everything with me.

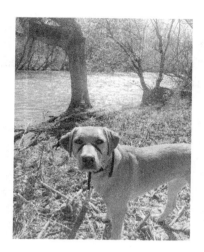
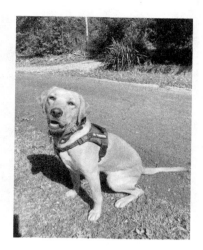

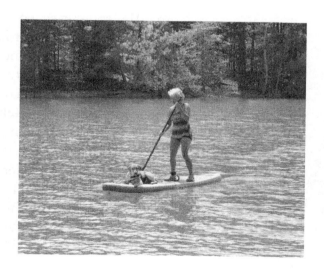

Tumor Effects on My Appearance:

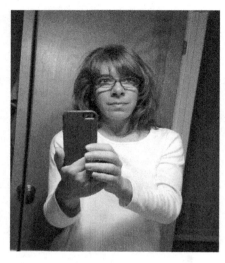

A random picture of me in 2012. This was around one year after finding the tumor.

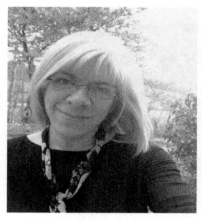

In 2018, roughly seven years after the tumor was first found. So, from 2011 to the time of this picture in 2018, the tumor had been producing IGF-1 for roughly seven years. I felt like my features were changing, but it made no sense to me. My nose, face, and jaw were wider, and my tongue was bigger. I honestly thought it had something to do with my diet. You know, when you eat that piece of cake, chocolate bar, and ice cream and wonder how it will affect you. That's kind of how I was feeling.

Dan, Violet, and me almost six months post-surgery. I was told that tissue growth and swelling would go down, but bone growth would stay the same. I think my face has slimmed down a little. I know my hands and feet have because I had since put on a pair of old sandals and they were too big!

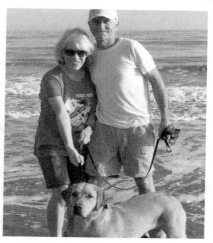

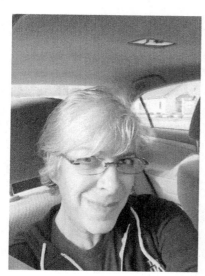

In May 2021, almost one year post-surgery. I felt like the swelling tissue changes, particularly in my face, had decreased some. I am on the road to recovery and things will take time, but I am so thankful and blessed.

My Family, My Life

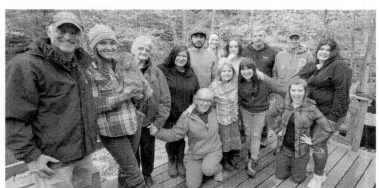

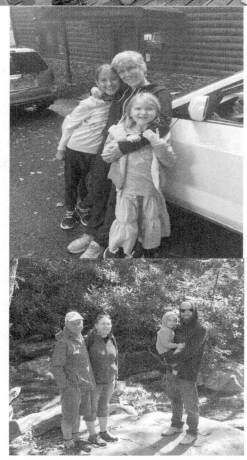

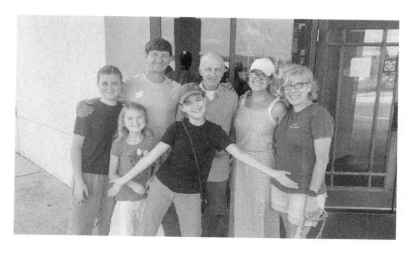

My passion for skiing keeps me going.

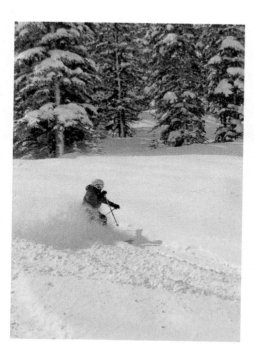

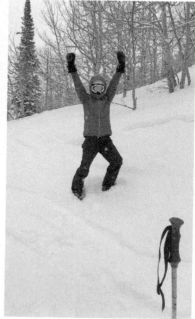